T0185629

Bariatric Psychology and Psychiatry

Alfonso Troisi

Bariatric Psychology and Psychiatry

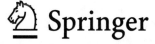 Springer

Alfonso Troisi
International Medical School
University of Rome Tor Vergata
Rome
Italy

ISBN 978-3-030-44836-3   ISBN 978-3-030-44834-9   (eBook)
https://doi.org/10.1007/978-3-030-44834-9

This Springer imprint is published by the registered company Springer Nature Switzerland AG
The registered company address is: Gewerbestrasse 11, 6330 Cham, Switzerland

*This book is dedicated to AS Roma 1927,
one of the greatest loves of my life.*

Preface

This is a book written for clinicians by a clinician. The importance of mental health assessment and care of bariatric patients has clearly emerged in the last decade. Yet, in most bariatric programs, the role of psychologists and psychiatrists is still marginal or poorly defined. In my opinion, one possible reason is that surgery is a medical branch more distant from psychology and psychiatry than any other clinical discipline. The mechanistic and systematic approach of surgery does not match well with the fluid concepts of psychology and psychiatry that are based on heterogeneous theoretical models, questionable diagnostic categories, and disputed treatment strategies.

The primary aim of this book is to foster communication between bariatric surgeons and mental health professionals. Optimal care of bariatric patients requires that each member of the clinical team understands the meaning and relevance of the data that are being collected during the preoperative and postoperative stages of assessment and treatment. Mental health reports should not be conceived of as separate pieces of clinical information that can be decrypted only by psychologists and psychiatrists. For this reason, each chapter includes basic notions on psychological constructs and psychiatric conditions that are easy to understand and memorize even if the reader has no training or education in the field of mental health. In sum, this is not a book written exclusively for bariatric psychologists and psychiatrists, although I hope that my colleagues in the field of mental health may benefit from the systematic review of data and clear indications of how to assist bariatric patients through their "surgical journey."

Bariatric psychology and psychiatry are rapidly evolving fields, and this implies that much of the data and indications reported in the book will be revised in the near future. In addition, it is likely that some parts reflect my personal opinions not shared by other mental health professionals. It would be great if the book could become the starting point for an open forum on current and future status of bariatric psychology and psychiatry. Feedback from readers is welcome.

Rome, Italy   Alfonso Troisi
April, 2020

Acknowledgements

My interest for bariatric psychology and psychiatry dates back to 15 years ago when I was involved in the psychosocial evaluation and psychiatric screening of patients referred to the bariatric unit of the University of Rome La Sapienza directed by Professor Nicola Basso, MD, President Emeritus of the *Società Italiana di Chirurgia dell'Obesità e delle Malattie Metaboliche* (SICOB).

The long-standing clinical and research collaboration with Professor Basso and his coworkers Professor Giovanni Casella, MD, and Professor Alfredo Genco, MD, has allowed me to interview more than 800 patients undergoing bariatric surgery and to learn the importance of the emerging disciplines of bariatric psychology and psychiatry. To all of them, I owe my sincere gratitude.

I wish to thank Catherine Mazars who, as Editor at Springer, welcomed this volume into the Springer clinical medicine books program. My deep gratitude to Dr. Roberta Croce Nanni, PsyD, for her advice in selecting the psychometric instruments and psychotherapeutic techniques that are most useful in assessing and treating bariatric patients.

Outline of the Book

Chapter 1: Bariatric Surgery and Mental Health

Chapter 1 explains the concepts of bariatric psychology and psychiatry, their relevance in contemporary bariatric surgery, and reasons to include psychologists and psychiatrists in multidisciplinary teams taking care of bariatric patients. This chapter and the following ones include graphical aids using a bullet point format, making assessment tips and key points easy to identify.

Chapters 2–5: Bariatric Psychology

These chapter provide an overview of the aspects of mental health that are investigated by bariatric psychology. The suite of psychological processes analyzed in these chapters plays a major role in influencing patients' perception of the outcomes of bariatric surgery and in determining their commitment to lifestyle changes and follow-up programs.

Chapters 6–14: Bariatric Psychiatry

These chapter present a detailed overview of the psychiatric conditions that are common among bariatric candidates or that may complicate post-surgery course. For each condition, the following areas will be discussed:

- Basic notions on definition, clinical features, and epidemiology.
- Diagnosis and assessment procedures including interviews and psychometric questionnaires.
- Data from studies of bariatric patients conducted before and after surgery. The focus is on the impact of the psychiatric condition on bariatric surgery outcomes (weight loss, weight regain, quality of life) and the impact of surgery on its course (remission, worsening, de novo onset).
- Clinical management of the condition including psychotherapy and/or psychopharmacology.

Chapter 15: Current Problems and Future Directions

This chapter provides an overview of unsolved issues in the clinical practice of bariatric psychology and psychiatry and of emerging research findings that are likely to change assessment and care of bariatric patients' mental health in the near future.

Appendix: Assessment Toolbox

Summary list of interview formats and psychometric questionnaires for assessing bariatric patients' mental health is provided in the Appendix. It also includes a selected list for basic assessment based on my clinical experience with bariatric patients.

Contents

Bariatric Surgery and Mental Health

Abstract

The popularity of bariatric surgery is growing at an impressive rate among both clinicians and patients with obesity. No other branch of surgery is so strictly intertwined with psychology and psychiatry as bariatric surgery. The study of mental health in bariatric patients has now reached a notable level of complexity as shown by the emergence of two distinct subspecialties. Bariatric psychology deals with normal individual differences in cognitive and emotional functioning that may impact patients' mental well-being before and after surgery. Bariatric psychiatry deals with the diagnosis and management of psychopathological conditions that deny or defer clearance for surgery, require pre-operative treatment, and worsen or emerge de novo after surgery. Initially, the scope of bariatric psychology and psychiatry was very limited. Goals included the discovery of weight loss predictors and the identification of those disordered behaviors and psychiatric symptoms that could put patients at risk for post-surgery complications. Now, goals are much more comprehensive and include changes in psychosocial and functional status. The field is moving toward an individually tailored definition of bariatric surgery success.

Keywords

Bariatric surgery · Mental health · Bariatric psychology · Bariatric psychiatry
Pre-surgery assessment · Post-surgery follow-up

© Springer Nature Switzerland AG 2020
A. Troisi, *Bariatric Psychology and Psychiatry*,
https://doi.org/10.1007/978-3-030-44834-9_1

1.1   Background

Bariatric surgery is the branch of surgery aimed at helping a person with obesity lose weight. Unlike alternative treatments (e.g., diet, exercise, behavior modifications, and weight loss medications), bariatric surgery is a reliable procedure for obtaining significant and long-lasting weight loss, up to 30% of total body weight (Shanti and Patel 2019). In addition, there is evidence that bariatric surgery can improve metabolic complications associated with obesity (e.g., type 2 diabetes) and therefore some documents refer to it as "weight and metabolic surgery." The popularity of bariatric surgery is growing at an impressive rate among both clinicians and patients with obesity. The data reported by the American Society for Metabolic and Bariatric Surgery (ASMBS) (https://asmbs. org/resources/estimate-of-bariatric-surgery-numbers, accessed 03 Jan 2020) show that, in the years between 2011 and 2018, the number of patients who underwent weight loss surgery in the United States rose from 158,000 to 252,000.

No other branch of surgery is so strictly intertwined with psychology and psychiatry as bariatric surgery. The changes engendered by bariatric surgery are not limited to rapid and significant weight loss. In the months and years following surgery, patients experience major modifications in their body image, day-to-day functioning, and social relationships. As a consequence, psychological adjustment is an integral component of the post-operative process, leading to successful outcomes. Bariatric surgery can impact mental health, for better but also for worse. In a cohort study of 24,766 patients who underwent bariatric surgery, over a 10-year study period, one out of six participants (16.7%) made at least one visit to a mental health service. Compared with before surgery, outpatient, emergency department, and inpatient psychiatric presentations were all significantly more common after surgery (Morgan et al. 2019). In the authors' interpretation, their findings suggest that the current guidelines recommending pre-operative psychological assessment and the postponement of surgery in patients with active psychiatric conditions may be either ineffectual or inconsistently adhered to.

The study of mental health in bariatric patients has now reached a notable level of complexity as shown by the emergence of two distinct subspecialties. Bariatric psychology deals with normal individual differences in cognitive and emotional functioning that may impact patients' mental well-being before and after surgery. Bariatric psychiatry deals with the diagnosis and management of psychopathological conditions that deny or defer clearance for surgery, require pre-operative treatment, and worsen or emerge de novo after surgery (Fig. 1.1).

This introductory chapter is organized as follows. A brief summary of the surgical procedures currently used is offered as basic information for mental health professionals who are not familiar with the latest developments of bariatric surgery. The subsequent sections address the 4 W's of bariatric psychology and psychiatry, that is, the four questions that inform mental health assessment and treatment of bariatric patients.

Fig. 1.1 Integration of bariatric psychology and bariatric psychiatry in defining the evolving goals of pre- and post-operative assessment of bariatric patients

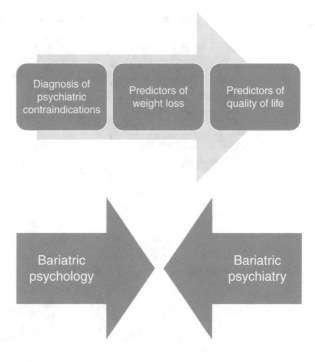

1.2   Types of Bariatric Surgery

There are two main types of surgery, almost always done via laparoscopic surgery: one that restricts how much can be eaten (restrictive) and one that limits absorption from the gut (malabsorptive) (Fig. 1.2). The most commonly performed procedures are sleeve gastrectomy and Roux-en-Y gastric bypass (RYGB). Biliopancreatic diversion, with or without duodenal switch, is less commonly performed but is often considered in extremely obese individuals. Other techniques are the adjustable gastric banding and intragastric balloons. Revision weight loss surgery is a surgical procedure that is performed on patients who have already undergone a form of bariatric surgery and have either had complications from such surgery or have not successfully achieved significant weight loss results from the initial surgery. The relative percentages in the United States for the year 2018 were: sleeve gastrectomy 61.4%, RYGB 17.0%, revision 15.4%, adjustable gastric banding 1.1%, and biliopancreatic diversion with duodenal switch 0.8% (https://asmbs.org/resources/estimate-of-bariatric-surgery-numbers). In the last 5 years, sleeve gastrectomy has continued to trend upward, while the Roux-en-Y gastric bypass and adjustable gastric banding have trended downward.

Sleeve gastrectomy is performed by placing an orogastric tube (approximately 12 mm diameter) along the lesser curve of the stomach and resecting the extra stomach. Although many regard sleeve gastrectomy as a restrictive procedure, it is increasingly recognized as a metabolic procedure. RYGB consists in restricting

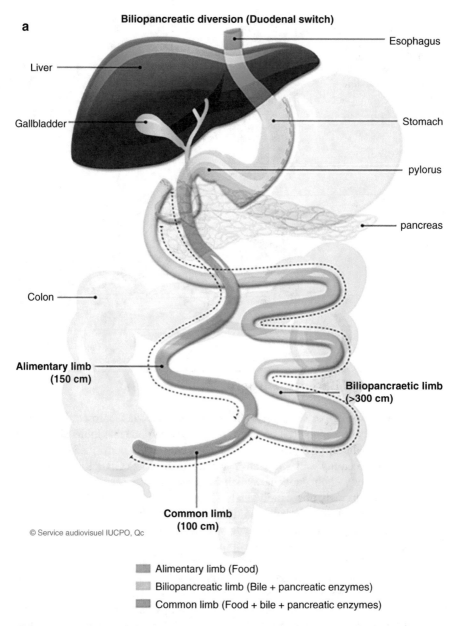

a   **Biliopancreatic diversion (Duodenal switch)**

Esophagus

Liver

Gallbladder

Stomach

pylorus

pancreas

Colon

Alimentary limb
(150 cm)

Biliopancraetic limb
(>300 cm)

Common limb
(100 cm)

© Service audiovisuel IUCPO, Qc

Alimentary limb (Food)

Biliopancreatic limb (Bile + pancreatic enzymes)

Common limb (Food + bile + pancreatic enzymes)

Fig. 1.2 (**a**) Duodenal switch, from Blaye-Felice S, Lebel S, Marceau S, Julien F, Biertho L. Duodenal switch. In: Lutfi R, Palermo M, Cadière G-B, editors, Global bariatric surgery. © Springer International Publishing AG; 2018. pp 113–24, with permission. (**b**) Roux-en-Y gastric bypass, from Mathus-Vliegen EMH, Dargent J, Bariatric surgery. © Springer International Publishing AG; 2018. pp 177–220, with permission. (**c**) Laparoscopic adjustable gastric banding, from Mathus-Vliegen EMH, Dargent J. Bariatric surgery. © Springer International Publishing AG; 2018. pp 177–220, with permission. (**d**) Sleeve gastrectomy, from Mathus-Vliegen EMH, Dargent J. Bariatric surgery. © Springer International Publishing AG; 2018. pp 177–220, with permission

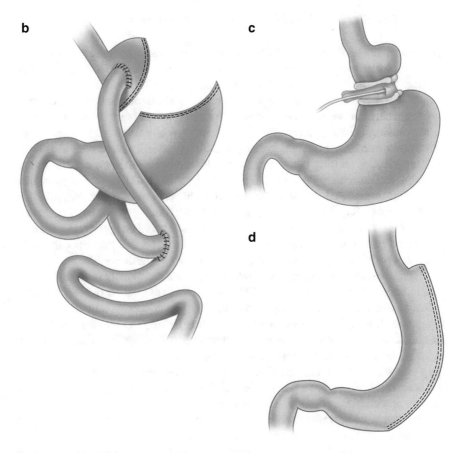

Fig. 1.2 (continued)

gastric volume to a 15–30 mL pouch, rerouting nutrient flow from the stomach into the proximal jejunum. RYGB reduces the absorption of food by excluding most of the stomach, duodenum, and upper intestine. Biliopancreatic diversion with duodenal switch creates a smaller tubular stomach pouch by removing part of the stomach with a segment of the small intestine anastomosed to the newly created stomach pouch, with three-fourths of the small intestine bypassed in this procedure. This type of surgery reduces the absorption of fat and induces changes in gut hormones that reduce appetite and improve satiety. In biliopancreatic diversion without duodenal switch, a vertical sleeve gastrectomy is constructed and the division of the duodenum is performed immediately beyond the pylorus. The alimentary limb is connected to the duodenum, whereas the iliopancreatic limb is anastomosed to the ileum 75 cm proximal to the ileocecal valve. In adjustable gastric banding, a band with an inner inflatable silastic balloon is placed around the proximal stomach just below the gastroesophageal junction. The band can be tightened through a subcutaneous access port by the injection or withdrawal of a saline solution.

1.3   The First W: Why Mental Health Assessment?

There are many reasons that explain why psychological and psychiatric assessments are an essential part of the clinical examination of bariatric patients. Unlike non-surgical treatments of obesity (e.g., diet, exercise, behavior modifications, and weight loss medications) for which risks are low and discontinuation can occur at any time, bariatric surgery has inherent risks and requires highly restrictive, long-term behavioral changes afterward. Patients are typically faced with initial dietary restrictions, permanent changes in eating and dietary habits, altered body sensations and experiences, shifting body image and self-care behaviors, new cognitions and feelings, and an emerging and different lifestyle. In addition, they may realize sometimes unexpected and significant changes in relationships that may result in marked stress (Snyder 2009). Thus, psychological and psychiatric assessments should serve not only as a gatekeeping measure but also as an opportunity for education and planning. It is during pre-operative interviews that patients can understand that bariatric surgery is only the first step toward a healthier life.

Another reason for mental health assessment is the complexity of informed consent in bariatric surgery (Wee et al. 2009). Clinicians are frequently unaware of the extent to which they communicate with jargon or use concepts that patients do not comprehend. In light of the decision that patients undergoing bariatric surgery are making when they consent to surgery, a thorough understanding of what they are agreeing to is essential. Patients should be able to articulate their rationale for surgery and why it is right at this time in their life. The evaluating clinician should ascertain if the patient has a good understanding: (1) of the nature and mechanics of surgery as well as the possible risks and complications of the procedure; (2) of what is expected post-operatively, including diet, exercise, follow-up, support group attendance, etc. If patients are unable to demonstrate a basic and clear understanding of these factors, they are referred back to the surgeon and/or nutritionist for additional counseling. A teach-to-goal educational approach, in which patient comprehension is evaluated and education continued until the patient exhibits mastery of the content, can help people with health limited literacy.

As said earlier, recent developments in the fields of bariatric psychology and psychiatry suggest that detection of psychiatric symptoms and diagnosis of psychiatric syndromes are not the only goals of mental health assessment. Yet, a primary function of the clinical evaluation still remains to uncover the presence of any psychiatric conditions that would impair the patient's ability to handle the surgery and to avoid post-surgery poor outcomes. Psychiatric disorders are common among bariatric patients. For example, Dawes et al. (2016) published a meta-analysis of 59 studies reporting the pre-operative prevalence of mental health conditions in 65,363 bariatric candidates. The three most common individual diagnoses, based on random-effects estimates of prevalence, were depression (19%), binge eating disorder (17%), and anxiety (12%). If lifetime, instead of current, prevalence rates are reported, about two-thirds of bariatric patients have a history of psychiatric disorders (Kalarchian et al. 2007). These findings, combined with those of Morgan et al. (2019) on the use of mental health services after surgery (see above), dictate a further reason why psychological and psychiatric assessments are indispensable.

1.4   The Second (Twofold) W: Who Should Evaluate Whom?

The growing awareness of the importance of mental health assessment brings consequences for the professional qualifications of those who evaluate bariatric patients. Some current bariatric programs still provide unclear information in this regard. Yet, as early as 2004, the ASBS published a document reporting detailed suggestions: *ASBS believes that the application and interpretation of objective tests, the ability to identify discrete risk factors not amenable to testing, and the capacity to conduct pertinent clinical interviews and to organize this information in a way that directly speaks to the adjustment of the individual after surgery require a particular level and kind of experience that is specific to bariatric surgery.* The document speaks explicitly of "clinicians": *It is also expected that evaluating clinicians hold a professional license that authorizes them to formulate a clinical diagnosis according to DSM-IV criteria. Additionally, their license should authorize them to conduct psychological evaluations, perform psychotherapy or counseling of adults with an Axis I or Axis II clinical diagnosis or other psychological conditions that may be a focus of clinical attention as outlined in the DSM-IV, and administer and interpret psychological tests … Finally, clinicians should have a level of expertise that allows them to develop clinical strategies for enhancing patient adherence to treatment (self-management) guidelines over the long-term course of post-operative care, develop relapse prevention strategies, and teach or facilitate life skills (e.g., modulating emotions, pacing oneself, and limit-setting) associated with using the surgical pouch and managing the disease of morbid obesity.* (https://asmbs.org/app/uploads/2014/05/PsychPreSurgicalAssessment.pdf, p. 15). Apart from minor differences (e.g., current diagnoses are based on DSM-5 criteria), the ASBS document is still a benchmark for setting the professional qualification of evaluators. In the future, it is likely that a specific training will be required to qualify as bariatric psychologist or bariatric psychiatrist.

The answer to the second W question (Which bariatric patients should be evaluated?) is much simpler: everyone. The belief that mental health assessment should be limited only to those candidates who report current psychiatric symptoms and/or a history of psychiatric disorders is unwarranted. The scope of mental health assessment is so wide (see the next section) that everyone seeking surgical treatment for obesity can benefit from it.

1.5   The Third W: What Should Be Assessed?

Assessment content includes topics that fall into the domains of either bariatric psychology or bariatric psychiatry. Although not always sharp enough, such a distinction is useful for organizing data collection. Psychosocial assessment focuses on patients' motivations, expectations, and post-surgery experiences; the understanding of surgery mechanics and necessary lifestyle changes; the capacity to adhere to pre- and post-operative regimens; eating habits and dietary preferences; physical activity and inactivity; personality traits with particular reference to coping skills and emotional processing; social support; body image and self-esteem; history of trauma/abuse; quality of life. Psychiatric assessment investigates current and/or past presence of psychopathological conditions, especially those that are more common in bariatric patients: eating disorders, depression, and anxiety. Bipolar and psychotic disorders are less common but deserve accurate diagnostic investigation because of their potential severity. Special attention should be devoted to symptoms of personality disorders, substance misuse, and cognitive impairment. Finally, suicidal ideation and suicidal behavior merit utmost consideration because of recent data showing increased suicide risk after bariatric surgery.

Despite the rising involvement of mental health professionals in bariatric surgery, little data exists on how to best evaluate these patients, and there are no uniform guidelines for the psychological and psychiatric assessment of surgery candidates. One point of general agreement is that the best strategy for data collection should include a combination of face-to-face interviews with the administration of validated psychometric instruments. Based on the topic under investigation, each chapter of this book provides some suggestions about the questionnaires that can be used. As for clinical interviews, one possible format is based on open-ended questions focusing on each of the topics outlined above and asked by a psychologist or a psychiatrist with extensive experience in the fields of obesity, eating disorders, and bariatric screening. It is much better if the evaluator is on staff or affiliated with the bariatric center. Such an integration can facilitate communication, maintain the support network, and provide continuity of care. Open-ended interviews have the advantage of lessening patients' sensation that they are being examined just to exclude the presence of psychiatric contraindications. Bariatric candidates face a unique situation when being evaluated by mental health professionals prior to surgery. They doubtlessly recognize the possibility of being denied surgery based on the evaluation and thus have an incentive to try to present themselves in as favorable a light as possible.

Open-ended interviews have a major drawback, however. A number of studies have demonstrated disagreement between results obtained from structured interviews (which are better for diagnosing psychopathology) and general clinical evaluations (Mitchell et al. 2010). A possible tradeoff between lessening patients' diffidence and collecting reliable clinical information is to divide data gathering into separate sessions, with the initial open-ended interview focusing on less thorny themes such as weight and diet history, motivations and expectations, quality of life, and social support.

Currently, there are two instruments that have been designed specifically for bariatric patients: The *PsyBari* (Mahony 2011) and the *Boston Interview* (Sogg and Mori 2008, 2009). The *PsyBari* is a paper-and-pencil psychological test designed specifically for pre-surgery psychological assessments. It includes a demographic section where patients record their medical, weight, diet, substance, and alcohol use histories and 115 items scored on a Likert scale. The *PsyBari* includes 11 subscales that measure constructs that are important in pre-surgical psychological evaluations. One of the subscales (the *Faking Good/Minimization/Denial Scale*) is designed to measure test taking response biases by assessing a patient's awareness of and willingness to acknowledge commonly reported behaviors and/or psychological states related to obesity. The scale consists of items that are endorsed positively by most patients (e.g., *It's hard to stay away from food that I really like*). Patients who respond negatively to these items are considered to be unaware of or unwilling to acknowledge common behaviors and/or psychological states related to obesity. The *Boston Interview* is a semi-structured interview protocol designed to collect information into seven major areas of assessment: (1) weight, diet, and nutrition history; (2) current eating behaviors; (3) medical history; (4) understanding of surgical procedures, risks, and the post-surgical regimen; (5) motivation and expectations of surgical outcome; (6) relationships and support system; and (7) psychiatric functioning. According to the authors, the standardized format offers two important advantages. First, the interview incorporates opportunities for patients to learn more about the procedure, allowing them to make more informed treatment decisions. Second, the standardized nature of the interview allows it to function as a useful tool for the collection of data to be used for research.

Finally, there is a relatively neglected topic that should be investigated during mental health assessment: the interaction between bariatric surgery and psychopharmacology. The scarce attention to this aspect in the literature is likely due to the uneven growth of bariatric psychology (well-developed) and bariatric psychiatry (still in infancy). Many bariatric patients use psychotropic drugs, especially antidepressants and anxiolytics. The reason is the high prevalence of depression and anxiety in this patient population. Bariatric surgery can exert different effects on medication regimen, including withdrawal of therapy because of post-surgery remission of symptoms and necessity to increase or decrease dosage because of altered pharmacokinetics (Monte et al. 2018). A system of close monitoring of patients that are undergoing bariatric surgery is required. This monitoring should include documentation of pre-surgery plasma levels of psychotropic drugs, periodic reassessment of the clinical picture to evaluate therapeutic efficacy and side effects, and measurements of plasma levels to determine the impact of surgery on drug pharmacokinetics (Roerig and Steffen 2015).

1.6   The Fourth W: When Should Assessment Be Made?

The outdated view that mental health assessment should serve exclusively as a gatekeeping measure implied the period just before surgery as the right time for evaluating bariatric patients. Nowadays, there is much evidence that periodic monitoring after surgery is as much or even more important than pre-surgery assessment (Rutledge et al. 2019). In most patients, the first year after surgery is associated with substantial weight loss and improvement in mental well-being. However, this "honeymoon" phase is sometimes followed by emerging problems including weight regain and emotional distress. Patients' subjective experiences may change over time, with major differences between early and later years after surgery. Using data from the Longitudinal Assessment of Bariatric Surgery (LABS) study, King et al. (2018) found that, in patients who underwent RYGB and achieved nadir weight, mental health–related quality of life declined in 27.7% of participants during the first year after nadir weight, with a 12.4% decline in satisfaction with surgery.

How long should periodic monitoring be extended after surgery? Understandably, bariatric patients may be less motivated to attend psychological and psychiatric evaluations when many years have elapsed since surgery. Yet, the few long-term longitudinal data that have been published so far show that patients may need help just when they are exiting the radar range of post-surgery surveillance. The study by Morgan et al. (2019) showing an increased utilization of mental health services after surgery covered a follow-up period of 10 years. The small study of Canetti et al. (2016) comparing bariatric patients with participants in a dietary program over a 10-year post-surgery period found that the surgery group achieved successful weight loss outcomes (27% reduction of pre-operative weight) and better than baseline health-related quality-of-life scores. However, their general mental health, neuroticism, sense of control, and fear of intimacy scores showed significant deterioration in comparison to pre-operative levels after 10 years. The dietary group participants remained psychologically stable among all three points in time. Likewise, Galli et al. (2018) reported significant impairment in patients' quality of life 10 years after biliointestinal bypass surgery in spite of substantial improvement of medical comorbidities. Thus, the answer to the question "How long should periodic monitoring be extended after surgery?" is: the longer the better.

1.7   Conclusion

The evolving status of the relationship between bariatric surgery and mental health implies an apparent paradox. On the one hand, there is growing evidence that pre-operative psychological evaluations exclude few patients and that conditions previously considered as psychiatric contraindications are now viewed as compatible with surgery clearance (Rutledge et al. 2019). This might suggest that mental health assessment is now less important than in the past. On the other hand, long-term longitudinal data show that bariatric surgery can be associated with increased post-operative risk for poorer quality of life, substance misuse, and suicide (Li and Wu 2016; Castaneda et al. 2019). This might suggest that mental health assessment is now more important than in the past.

The explanation for the paradox lies with the different goals of mental health assessment now and in the past. Initially, the scope of bariatric psychology and psychiatry was very limited. Goals included the discovery of weight loss predictors and the identification of those disordered behaviors and psychiatric symptoms that could put patients at risk for post-surgery complications. Now, goals are much more comprehensive and include changes in psychosocial and functional status. The field is moving toward an individually tailored definition of bariatric surgery success.

References

Canetti L, Bachar E, Bonne O. Deterioration of mental health in bariatric surgery after 10 years despite successful weight loss. Eur J Clin Nutr. 2016;70(1):17–22. Epub 2015 Jul 22. PubMed PMID: 26197876. https://doi.org/10.1038/ejcn.2015.112.

Castaneda D, Popov VB, Wander P, Thompson CC. Risk of suicide and self-harm is increased after bariatric surgery—a systematic review and meta-analysis. Obes Surg. 2019;29(1):322–33. Review. PubMed PMID: 30343409. https://doi.org/10.1007/s11695-018-3493-4.

Dawes AJ, Maggard-Gibbons M, Maher AR, Booth MJ, Miake-Lye I, Beroes JM, Shekelle PG. Mental health conditions among patients seeking and undergoing bariatric surgery: a meta-analysis. JAMA. 2016;315(2):150–63. PubMed PMID: 26757464. https://doi.org/10.1001/jama.2015.18118.

Galli F, Cavicchioli M, Vegni E, Panizzo V, Giovanelli A, Pontiroli AE, Micheletto G. Ten years after bariatric surgery: bad quality of life promotes the need of psychological interventions. Front Psychol. 2018;9:2282. eCollection 2018. PubMed PMID: 30524346; PubMed Central PMCID: PMC6262042. https://doi.org/10.3389/fpsyg.2018.02282.

Kalarchian MA, Marcus MD, Levine MD, Courcoulas AP, Pilkonis PA, Ringham RM, Soulakova JN, Weissfeld LA, Rofey DL. Psychiatric disorders among bariatric surgery candidates: relationship to obesity and functional health status. Am J Psychiatry. 2007;164(2):328–34; quiz 374. PubMed PMID: 17267797.

King WC, Hinerman AS, Belle SH, Wahed AS, Courcoulas AP. Comparison of the performance of common measures of weight regain after bariatric surgery for association with clinical outcomes. JAMA. 2018;320(15):1560–9. PubMed PMID: 30326125; PubMed Central PMCID: PMC6233795. https://doi.org/10.1001/jama.2018.14433.

Li L, Wu LT. Substance use after bariatric surgery: a review. J Psychiatr Res. 2016;76:16–29. Epub 2016 Jan 22. Review. PubMed PMID: 26871733; PubMed Central PMCID: PMC4789154. https://doi.org/10.1016/j.jpsychires.2016.01.009.

Mahony D. Psychological assessments of bariatric surgery patients. Development, reliability, and exploratory factor analysis of the PsyBari. Obes Surg. 2011;21(9):1395–406. PubMed PMID: 20306154. https://doi.org/10.1007/s11695-010-0108-0.

Mitchell JE, Steffen KJ, de Zwaan M, Ertelt TW, Marino JM, Mueller A. Congruence between clinical and research-based psychiatric assessment in bariatric surgical candidates. Surg Obes Relat Dis. 2010;6(6):628–34. Epub 2010 Feb 6. PubMed PMID: 20727837; PubMed Central PMCID: PMC3854936. https://doi.org/10.1016/j.soard.2010.01.007.

Monte SV, Russo KM, Mustafa E, Caruana JA. Impact of sleeve gastrectomy on psychiatric medication use and symptoms. J Obes. 2018;2018:8532602. eCollection 2018. PubMed PMID: 30410796; PubMed Central PMCID: PMC6205308. https://doi.org/10.1155/2018/8532602.

Morgan DJR, Ho KM, Platell C. Incidence and determinants of mental health service use after bariatric surgery. JAMA Psychiat. 2019. [Epub ahead of print] PubMed PMID: 31553420; PubMed Central PMCID: PMC6763981. https://doi.org/10.1001/jamapsychiatry.2019.2741.

Roerig JL, Steffen K. Psychopharmacology and bariatric surgery. Eur Eat Disord Rev. 2015;23(6):463–9. Epub 2015 Sep 3. Review. PubMed PMID: 26338011. https://doi.org/10.1002/erv.2396.

Rutledge T, Ellison JK, Phillips AS. Revising the bariatric psychological evaluation to improve clinical and research utility. J Behav Med. 2019. [Epub ahead of print] PubMed PMID: 31127435. https://doi.org/10.1007/s10865-019-00060-1.

Shanti H, Patel AG. Surgery for obesity. Medicine. 2019;47(3):184–7. ISSN 1357-3039. https://doi.org/10.1016/j.mpmed.2018.12.011.

Snyder AG. Psychological assessment of the patient undergoing bariatric surgery. Ochsner J. 2009;9(3):144–8. PubMed PMID: 21603431; PubMed Central PMCID: PMC3096263.

Sogg S, Mori DL. Revising the Boston Interview: incorporating new knowledge and experience. Surg Obes Relat Dis. 2008;4(3):455–63. Epub 2008 Apr 23. Review. PubMed PMID: 18436484. https://doi.org/10.1016/j.soard.2008.01.007.

Sogg S, Mori DL. Psychosocial evaluation for bariatric surgery: the Boston interview and opportunities for intervention. Obes Surg. 2009;19(3):369–77. Epub 2008 Sep 16. Review. PubMed PMID: 18795379. https://doi.org/10.1007/s11695-008-9676-7.

Wee CC, Pratt JS, Fanelli R, Samour PQ, Trainor LS, Paasche-Orlow MK. Best practice updates for informed consent and patient education in weight loss surgery. Obesity (Silver Spring). 2009;17(5):885–8. Epub 2009 Feb 19. PubMed PMID: 19396067. https://doi.org/10.1038/oby.2008.567.

Patients' Motivations, Expectations, and Experiences

2

Abstract

One of the tasks of mental health professionals who take care of bariatric patients is to analyze the motivations that lead the patient to seek surgery treatment for obesity, the entire spectrum of changes the patient expects to see as a result of undergoing surgery, and the patient's long-term experiences after bariatric surgery. Patients' motivations, expectations, and experiences play an important role in determining if bariatric surgery is perceived by the individual patient as more or less successful. There are four main motivations driving patients to seek surgical treatment for obesity: health concerns, medical conditions, physical fitness, and appearance. Unrealistic expectations may cause poor satisfaction with surgery outcomes and lead to post-operative frustration, depression, and opposition to implement behavioral changes. Bariatric surgery is not a "magic bullet," and patients' unrealistic expectations should be discussed and amended during psychosocial assessment. A comprehensive assessment of short- and long-term outcomes of bariatric surgery goes far beyond just measuring weight loss and medical complications. Clinical objective measures should be integrated with patients' subjective experiences of the impact of surgery on a variety of domains (e.g., eating behavior, body image, psychological well-being, and quality of life).

Keywords

Motivations · Expectations · Experiences · Unrealistic goals · Quality of life

2.1 Background

Pontiroli et al. (2017) have conceptualized bariatric surgery as a voyage affecting patients' life for years. Such a description is very far from the idea that bariatric surgery is just a hit-and-run technical operation like many other surgical procedures.

As a voyage, bariatric surgery should be well prepared in advance, and the psychological processes preceding and following it should be explored thoroughly. One of the tasks of mental health professionals who take care of bariatric patients is to analyze such psychological processes, including the motivations that lead the patient to seek surgery treatment for obesity, the entire spectrum of changes the patient expects to see as a result of undergoing surgery, and the patient's long-term experiences after bariatric surgery. This chapter reviews published data on motivations, expectations, and experiences of bariatric patients and examines the best procedures to assess them through interviews and questionnaires.

2.2   Motivations

Based on published data, there are four main motivations driving patients to seek surgical treatment for obesity: health concerns, medical conditions, physical fitness, and appearance (Fig. 2.1). Libeton et al. (2004) assessed individuals' motivations for undergoing adjustable gastric band procedure. The participants were asked to rank a total of six statements (fitness, limitations, health, medical, appearance, embarrassment), in order from the most important reason to the least important reason for undergoing the surgery. The number one reason was health concerns (28.4%) followed by appearance (23.6%) and medical condition (23.6%). Women were more likely to select appearance as their top reason, whereas men were more likely to select medical condition. In the study of Wee et al. (2006), health reasons were selected as the most important factor for seeking

Fig. 2.1 The four main motivations driving patients to seek bariatric surgery. The relative importance of each motivation varies with the composition of the study sample (e.g., appearance is more important for women)

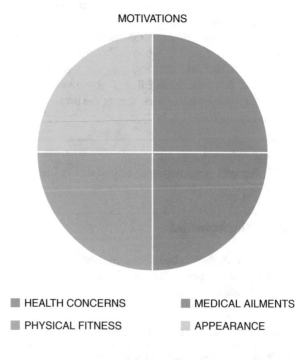

MOTIVATIONS

■ HEALTH CONCERNS   ■ MEDICAL AILMENTS

■ PHYSICAL FITNESS   APPEARANCE

bariatric surgery by 84% of the 44 participants. Munoz et al. (2007) asked an open-ended question (*Why are you seeking weight loss surgery?*) to 109 individuals seeking bariatric surgery. The order in which the participants wrote their responses were categorized by the authors as the individuals' first, second, and third reason for their desire to have bariatric surgery, and those reasons were then placed into categories to calculate percentages. The vast majority (73.4%) of respondents endorsed current medical ailments as their primary reason for seeking weight loss surgery. Patients who responded with a secondary reason for desiring surgery reported primarily psychological and quality of life reasons. In the study by Brantley et al. (2014), of the 360 participants, 187 (52%) rated health concerns (*I am concerned that my health will deteriorate and my life may be shortened*) as their number one reason for undergoing bariatric surgery. Medical conditions (*I want to improve medical conditions associated with my obesity*) was the second most commonly reported primary reason and functionality the third (fitness 5% and physical limitations 4%). Only 4% selected appearance as the primary reason. There were no significant gender differences.

The recent study by Peacock et al. (2018) analyzed the relationship between patients' motivations and surgery outcomes in a retrospective convenience sample of 345 participants recruited from an obesity support website to complete an online survey. Most participants reported a physical health–related motivation, but participants with greater perceived affective motivational responses cited prevention of death and viewing surgery as their last option to a higher extent. Participants with greater perceived affective response exhibited significantly better weight loss outcomes, indicating that some emotional component to motivation may improve long-term success.

2.3   Expectations

Not only clinicians but also patients know that bariatric surgery is the most effective weight loss treatment that currently exists. However, bariatric surgery is not a "magic bullet" and patients' unrealistic expectations should be discussed and amended during psychosocial assessment (Table 2.1). Unrealistic expectations may cause poor satisfaction with surgery outcomes and lead to post-operative frustration, depression and opposition to implement behavioral changes (Ghaferi and Varban 2018).

Opozda et al. (2018) analyzed pre-surgical expectations of eating behavior change in a sample of 206 Australian bariatric patients. Patients' expectations varied widely in terms of content and focus on realistic goals. The most common expectations were that surgery: (1) would help them eat less and feel increased satiety (*I want to be able to eat less and feel satisfied instead of constantly feeling hungry*); (2) would improve or cure disordered eating behaviors (*I expect to have a "round the clock" solution to prevent grazing and emotional eating*). A minority of patients had unrealistic expectations such as hopes that surgery would simply "fix" things including bad eating habits without personal effort. These findings confirm

Table 2.1 Unrealistic expectations that need to be discussed during pre-operative interviews

DOMAIN	UNREALISTIC GOAL
Weight loss	Surgery allows lose weight even if people will retain their current lifestyle habits.
Eating behavior	Maladaptive eating behaviors will disappear after surgery.
Medical comorbidities	Surgery will cure all medical comorbidities related to obesity.
Appearance	Surgery allows getting complete satisfaction with one's own new body image.
Physical fitness	Surgery by itself will guarantee an optimal level of physical fitness.
Emotional problems	Obesity is the cause of current emotional problems. Surgery is the definitive solution.

the importance of patients' education about the impact of different bariatric procedures on eating behavior. In particular, bariatric candidates should be aware that disordered eating behaviors and excessive hunger and appetite are not always cured or even improved by bariatric surgery, and that these difficulties may continue, worsen, or even begin de novo after surgery.

One major aspect to be discussed with patients when investigating their expectations is mental control over eating and lifestyle habits. Interviews with bariatric candidates suggest that they commonly believe that they have lost control over their own diet and ability to lose weight and feel that this control cannot be regained through personal effort. Choosing to undergo bariatric surgery is seen as a way to end the never-ending, unwinnable struggle with food and weight, and hand control over to a surgeon who will release them from obesity by changing how their body works (Opolski et al. 2015). Analyses of interview narratives indicate that some bariatric candidates are looking for a new bodily mechanism to help them control their eating, as they believe their mind is no longer able to do so. Such a passive attitude needs to be corrected. Patients should know that they have to play an active role in pre- and post-operative treatment and that changes to diet and physical activity are essential for successful outcomes. Pre-operative education should make it clear that the hope of retaining current lifestyle habits and still lose weight after surgery is unrealistic. Using the metaphor of bariatric surgery as a voyage (Pontiroli et al. 2017), patients should be said that without perseverance and diligence it is difficult to reach any destination.

The impact of surgery on interpersonal relationships is another issue that needs to be discussed. Most bariatric candidates report feeling stigmatized because of their weight, and many had received negative and judgmental comments from others (Homer et al. 2016). They describe long-standing shame and embarrassment regarding their appearance, day-to-day activities, and social functioning. Activities normal to others (e.g., parties, trips, and holidays) often cause anxiety and avoidance strategies. Therefore, patients expect surgery to improve not only their physical health but also their interpersonal relationships. Such an expectation is realistic considering that weight loss is generally associated with enhanced self-confidence, better mood, and improved mobility, which enable patients to do more activities with their partners and friends. However, even positive changes may imply new challenges. For example, patients sometimes report that their new body image and identity disrupt an entrenched dependency dynamic in romantic partnerships or close friendships. After losing weight, patients may become more assertive and more insistent in claiming their own needs, which may not be a welcome change for their family members or work colleagues. During pre-operative assessment, mental health professionals should encourage patients to reflect on the possible reactions of their significant others, and how they will manage new interpersonal challenges (Sogg 2012).

2.4   Experiences

A comprehensive assessment of short- and long-term outcomes of bariatric surgery goes far beyond just measuring weight loss and medical complications. Clinical objective measures should be integrated with patients' subjective experiences of the impact of surgery on a variety of domains (e.g., eating behavior, body image, psychological well-being, and quality of life).

The study by Opozda et al. (2018) quoted in the previous section reported on patients' experiences of changes in eating behavior after different bariatric procedures (i.e., adjustable gastric banding, AGB; vertical sleeve gastrectomy, VSG; Roux-en-Y gastric bypass, RYGB). The most commonly reported positive eating-related experience after all three procedures was eating less, followed by making better and more balanced choices about what, when, and how to eat. The proportion of patients reporting at least one positive eating-related experience did not significantly differ by procedure. Specific positive eating-related experiences also did not show any procedure-based variance. The proportions reporting at least one negative eating-related experience did not vary by procedure. However, differences were seen in the frequency of a number of specific experiences. Those in the VSG group more frequently reported experiencing little or no reduction in hunger after their surgery. Unhelpful or unwanted food intolerances, somatic reactions, or food preference changes were most commonly reported by those with AGB than other procedures. In each group, there was no difference in the proportions of patients reporting that their disordered eating behaviors had improved or resolved post-surgery (RYGB 15%, AGB 15%, and VSG 18%), and those who said their disordered eating had instead persisted or emerged de novo post-surgery (RYGB 15%, AGB 15%, and VSG 18%). Reports of negative eating-related experiences were more frequent after 18 months or more than 2–17.9 months post-surgery. A greater proportion of patients also noted that the positive changes they had experienced early-on had not persisted in the long run.

There is mounting evidence that patients' subjective experiences change over time, with major differences between early and later years after surgery. Using data from the Longitudinal Assessment of Bariatric Surgery (LABS) study, King et al. (2018) found that, in patients who underwent RYGB and achieved nadir weight, mental health–related quality of life declined in 27.7% of participants during the first year after nadir weight, with a 12.4% decline in satisfaction with surgery.

Studies that have investigated quality of life (QOL) in bariatric patients provide indirect information on their post-operative subjective experiences. QOL is a subjective assessment that can be determined only by the patient. Two patients with identical post-operative health status may have very different subjective assessment of their own QOL. Reported findings on QOL vary widely depending on the questionnaires used to measure it. There are generic instruments intended for general use, regardless of clinical condition, such the *Short Form-36* (SF-36) or the *Health Related Quality of Life Questionnaire* (HRQL). Other survey instruments have been designed for specific use in bariatric surgery such as the *Post-Bariatric Surgery Appearance Questionnaire* or the *Bariatric Analysis and Reporting Outcome System* (BAROS) (Mazer et al. 2017).

In spite of methodological problems with assessment procedures, some findings are consistent across the majority of studies (Hachem and Brennan 2016). QOL improves dramatically after surgery but then stabilizes at 1–2 years following surgery. This mirrors weight loss and comorbidity improvement suggesting that QOL improvements following bariatric surgery are at least in part attributed to weight loss. However, not all domains of QOL improve, and weight loss alone does not fully account for variations in QOL improvements following bariatric surgery. It is likely that other factors such as mental health and social support may contribute to QOL improvements. Physical functioning consistently improves following bariatric surgery, while few significant improvements are found in mental health and psychosocial functioning. This finding suggests that improvements in global QOL are most likely driven by a significant improvement in physical, but not mental, QOL. Based on these findings, Hachem and Brennan (2016) have concluded that there is: *a need for adjunctive interventions targeting mental health and social and environmental factors to facilitate improvement in all domains of QOL following bariatric surgery.* (p. 407).

Questionnaires and survey instruments are useful to collect data from large samples but only extended interviews and open-ended questions allow clinicians to gain perspective on the subjective experiences of bariatric patients. In the study by Perdue and Neil (2019) based on Herman's Dialogic Self Theory, fifty-five bariatric patients were asked to share their thoughts about their post-operative experience (18–30 months post-surgery) with the investigator. Individual responses were analyzed and divided into four dominant categories. The most common category was related to shopping and clothing. Within such a category, patients reported both positive experiences like "dream come true" (*I have always been a trendy dresser; now I can find more*) and negative experiences like "size disorientation" (*I went to a plus size store and was told by the clerk that their clothes would not fit me*). The second most common open-ended response category was about relationship transitions, both positive (*My family used to have to wait for me: now I can keep up*) and negative (*When I was fat, I was not a threat. But now that I am thinner, my girlfriends see me as a threat to their men*). The third category included responses that explained how surgery changed patients' focus on "the new body" ("*I never trusted my body before; now I will kayak and ride a roller coaster*"). The fourth category (*cheating on the fat person inside*) reflected patients' difficulty with the transition from an obese identity to a lower weight identity (*I look in the mirror and say, "Is that really me?"*). Interestingly, many of the participants stated that their recovery had a large psychological component for which they felt that they had not been fully prepared.

ASSESSMENT TIPS

Assess the motivations that lead the patient to seek surgery treatment for obesity.

Assess the entire spectrum of changes the patient expects to see as a result of undergoing surgery.

Assess the patient's subjective experiences throughout the different phases following surgery and weight loss.

Integrate survey instruments with openended questions.

2.5 Clinical Management

The goal of pre- and post-operative psychosocial assessment of bariatric patients goes well beyond to diagnose psychiatric conditions that can predict poor outcome or complicate recovery. The data reviewed in this chapter show that patients' motivations, expectations, and experiences play an important role in determining if bariatric surgery is perceived by the individual patient as more or less successful.

The pre-operative interview should include an exhaustive discussion of patients' motivations and expectations, with a special focus on unrealistic goals. To do that, the clinician should ascertain how much the patient knows about what is actually done in the surgical procedure of choice. To give a truly informed consent, the patient needs to know not only the risks and complications related to surgery but also the efforts required to change lifestyle habits. The post-operative assessment should explore the patient's subjective experiences throughout the different phases following surgery and weight loss. The clinician should ascertain if the patient is encountering problems with psychological adjustment to their new body identity and social role. However, the clinician should be aware that patients may have individual preferences regarding information to be discussed during pre-operative interviews.

Coblijn et al. (2018) showed that patients wished for information about the consequences of surgery on daily life, whereas the importance of information concerning complications decreased when their incidence lessened. In their sample of 112 bariatric candidates, patients deemed the opportunity to ask questions (96.4%) the most important feature of the consult, followed by a realistic view on expectations, for example, results of the procedure (95.5%) and information concerning the consequences of surgery for daily life (89.1%). Information about the risk of complications on the order of 10% was desired by 93% of patients; 48% desired information about lower risks (0.1%). Only 25 patients (22.3%) desired detailed information concerning their weight loss after surgery.

In conclusion, an optimal management of individualized pre- and post-operative treatment plans should be based on a comprehensive psychological profile of the bariatric patient that includes their motivations, expectations, and experiences. All these individual features interact with personal history, personality traits, and the possible presence of psychopathology in determining short- and long-term outcomes of bariatric surgery.

KEY POINTS

Unrealistic expectations may cause poor satisfaction with surgery outcomes.

Successful outcome depends in part on patients' pre-operative motivations and expectations, and post-surgery experiences.

Interventions targeting mental health and environmental factors facilitate improvement in all domains of quality of life following bariatric surgery.

References

Brantley PJ, Waldo K, Matthews-Ewald MR, Brock R, Champagne CM, Church T, Harris MN, McKnight T, McKnight M, Myers VH, Ryan DH. Why patients seek bariatric surgery: does insurance coverage matter? Obes Surg. 2014;24(6):961–4. PubMed PMID: 24671622; PubMed Central PMCID: PMC4111953. https://doi.org/10.1007/s11695-014-1237-7.

Coblijn UK, Lagarde SM, de Raaff CAL, van Wagensveld BA, Smets EMA. Patients' preferences for information in bariatric surgery. Surg Obes Relat Dis. 2018;14(5):665–73. Epub 2018 Jan 31. https://doi.org/10.1016/j.soard.2018.01.029.

Ghaferi AA, Varban OA. Setting appropriate expectations after bariatric surgery: evaluating weight regain and clinical outcomes. JAMA. 2018;320(15):1543–4. https://doi.org/10.1001/jama.2018.14241.

Hachem A, Brennan L. Quality of life outcomes of bariatric surgery: a systematic review. Obes Surg. 2016;26(2):395–409. Review.

Homer CV, Tod AM, Thompson AR, Allmark P, Goyder E. Expectations and patients' experiences of obesity prior to bariatric surgery: a qualitative study. BMJ Open. 2016;6(2):e009389. PubMed PMID: 26857104; PubMed Central PMCID: PMC4746450. https://doi.org/10.1136/bmjopen-2015-009389.

King WC, Hinerman AS, Belle SH, Wahed AS, Courcoulas AP. Comparison of the performance of common measures of weight regain after bariatric surgery for association with clinical outcomes. JAMA. 2018;320(15):1560–9. PubMed PMID: 30326125; PubMed Central PMCID: PMC6233795. https://doi.org/10.1001/jama.2018.14433.

Libeton M, Dixon JB, Laurie C, O'Brien PE. Patient motivation for bariatric surgery: characteristics and impact on outcomes. Obes Surg. 2004;14(3):392–8.

Mazer LM, Azagury DE, Morton JM. Quality of life after bariatric surgery. Curr Obes Rep. 2017;6(2):204–10. Review. https://doi.org/10.1007/s13679-017-0266-7.

Munoz DJ, Lal M, Chen EY, Mansour M, Fischer S, Roehrig M, Sanchez-Johnsen L, Dymek-Valenitine M, Alverdy J, le Grange D. Why patients seek bariatric surgery: a qualitative and quantitative analysis of patient motivation. Obes Surg. 2007;17(11):1487–91.

Opolski M, Chur-Hansen A, Wittert G. The eating-related behaviours, disorders and expectations of candidates for bariatric surgery. Clin Obes. 2015;5(4):165–97. Review. https://doi.org/10.1111/cob.12104.

Opozda M, Wittert G, Chur-Hansen A. Patients' expectations and experiences of eating behaviour change after bariatric procedures. Clin Obes. 2018;8(5):355–65. Epub 2018 Aug 16. https://doi.org/10.1111/cob.12273.

Peacock JC, Perry L, Morien K. Bariatric patients' reported motivations for surgery and their relationship to weight status and health. Surg Obes Relat Dis. 2018;14(1):39–45. Epub 2017 Oct 12. https://doi.org/10.1016/j.soard.2017.10.005.

Perdue TO, Neil JA. 'Shopping for a new body': descriptions of bariatric post-operative adjustment. Eat Weight Disord. 2019. [Epub ahead of print]. https://doi.org/10.1007/s40519-019-00783-9.

Pontiroli AE, Ceriani V, Folli F. Patients' expectations are important for success in bariatric surgery. Obes Surg. 2017;27(9):2469–70. https://doi.org/10.1007/s11695-017-2788-1.

Sogg S. Assessment of bariatric surgery candidates: the clinical interview. In: Mitchell JE, de Zwaan M, editors. Psychosocial assessment and treatment of bariatric surgery patients. New York, NY: Routledge; 2012. p. 15–36.

Wee CC, Jones DB, Davis RB, Bourland AC, Hamel MB. Understanding patients' value of weight loss and expectations for bariatric surgery. Obes Surg. 2006;16(4):496–500.

Personality Traits

3

Abstract

The assessment of personality traits is an important component of the psychosocial evaluation of bariatric patients for at least two different reasons. First, personality traits exert a major influence on a wide range of behaviors that make a difference between poor and good outcomes of surgery treatment for obesity. Second, compared to psychiatric symptoms, bariatric candidates' self-report information about personality traits is less subjected to conscious alteration because personality traits are perceived as not relevant for obtaining clearance to surgery. The pre-operative personality profile of patients with better surgery outcomes is a combination of high cooperativeness, high persistence, low novelty seeking, and low impulsivity. Additional and related predictors of good outcome are an internal locus of control, a low tendency toward externalizing behaviors, a secure attachment style, and low levels of alexithymia. Such a suite of personality traits modulates a variety of individual and social behaviors that are relevant to successful pre- and post-operative treatment plans including the capacity and willingness to modify dietary habits, to increase levels of routine physical activity, to restrain alcohol consumption, and to attend monitoring appointments.

Keywords

Personality · Temperament · Character · Impulsivity · Locus of control
Externalizing behavior · Attachment style · Alexithymia

3.1 Background

There is a striking discrepancy between the number of research papers (many) focusing on personality traits in patients seeking surgery treatment for obesity and the attention (little) dedicated to personality traits by clinical documents and

© Springer Nature Switzerland AG 2020   23
A. Troisi, *Bariatric Psychology and Psychiatry*,
https://doi.org/10.1007/978-3-030-44834-9_3

guidelines for the pre- and post-operative assessment of mental health in bariatric surgery. Two possible reasons are the complexity of personality assessment compared to the diagnosis of psychopathology and the prevalent orientation of contemporary clinical psychology and psychiatry toward the definition of categories instead of dimensions. Yet, neglecting personality traits deprives the evaluating clinician of a piece of information that can be very useful to predict and optimize the outcomes of bariatric surgery, as shown by the findings reported in the present chapter.

3.2   Basic Notions

Personality refers to individual differences in characteristic patterns of thinking, feeling, and behaving that become more stable from childhood to adulthood. These enduring patterns are described as personality traits or dimensions. There are many different ways to measure personality traits depending on the conceptual model of personality structure that informs the psychometric instruments to be used. In this chapter, the focus will be only on those personality traits that have been investigated in studies of bariatric patients: temperament and character, impulsivity, locus of control, internalizing and externalizing behaviors, attachment style, and alexithymia.

3.2.1   Temperament and Character

Cloninger's psychobiological model of personality identifies four dimensions of temperament (novelty seeking: the tendency to approach and be excited by novel stimuli; harm avoidance: the tendency to inhibit behavior and to experience anxiety in response to novel or potentially dangerous stimuli; persistence: the ability to maintain a behavior in favor of valued goals despite the lack of immediate reward; and reward dependence: responsiveness to social reward) and three dimensions of character (self-directedness: the ability to orient behavior according one's own goals; cooperativeness: the ability to successfully cooperate and get along with others; and self-transcendence; the ability to feel part of the world as a whole). The psychometric instrument derived from the Cloninger's model is the *Temperament and Character Inventory* (TCI-Revised).

3.2.2   Impulsivity

Impulsivity is a multidimensional concept that has been defined variously as an inability to wait, a tendency to act without forethought, insensitivity to consequences, and an inability to inhibit inappropriate behaviors. The *Barratt Impulsiveness Scale-11* (BIS-11) is a widely used and well-validated personality measure of impulsivity. It consists of 30 statements, which form six factors determined by principal-components analyses: attention, motor impulsivity (e.g., '*I do things without thinking*'), self-control, cognitive complexity (e.g., *I make up my mind quickly*), perseverance, and cognitive instability.

3.2.3   Locus of Control

Locus of control is an individual's belief system regarding the causes of his or her experiences and the factors to which that person attributes success or failure. This concept is usually divided into two categories: internal and external. A person with an external locus of control, who attributes his or her success to luck or fate, will be less likely to make the effort needed to change lifestyle habits. People with an external locus of control are also more likely to experience anxiety, frustration, and anger since they believe that they are not in control of their lives. Two widely used measures of locus of control are the *Multidimensional Health Locus of Control* (MHLC) and the *Weight Locus of Control* (WLOC).

3.2.4   Internalizing/Externalizing

The distinction between internalizing (indicating liability to experience anxiety and depression) and externalizing (indicating liability to experience substance misuse and antisocial behaviors) dimensions originated within child psychopathology research, but it has been subsequently applied to adults (Caspi and Moffitt 2018). Internalizing and externalizing scales are included in the *Minnesota Multiphasic Personality Inventory-Second Edition Restructured Form* (MMPI-2-RF).

3.2.5   Attachment Style

In the last two decades, attachment theory has become a prominent model for explaining personality processes and close relationships in adulthood. Basically, adult attachment styles reflect individual differences in attachment security. There are two dimensions of insecurity underlying all self-report measures of adult attachment. The first dimension, attachment-related anxiety, is concerned with a strong desire for closeness and protection, intense worries about abandonment, and the use of hyperactivating strategies to deal with attachment-related distress. People with high levels of attachment-related anxiety are said to have an insecure-anxious attachment style. The second dimension, attachment-related avoidance, is concerned with discomfort with closeness, preference for emotional distance and self-reliance, and the use of deactivating strategies to deal with attachment-related distress. People with high levels of attachment-related avoidance are said to have an insecure-avoidant attachment style. The most widely used self-report measures of adult attachment style are the *Relationship Questionnaire* (RQ), the *Attachment Style Questionnaire* (ASQ), and the *Experiences in Close Relationships* (ECR).

3.2.6 Alexithymia

Alexithymia is a personality trait describing individuals with deficits in emotion processing and awareness. Classically, alexithymia has been defined to comprise multiple facets including difficulty identifying and distinguishing emotions from bodily sensations, difficulty describing and verbalizing emotions, poverty of fantasy life, externally oriented thinking style, and poor empathizing. The *Toronto Alexithymia Scale* (TAS-20) is a self-rated alexithymia measure that captures three interrelated, core alexithymic features: difficulties identifying feelings, difficulties describing feelings, and concrete thinking. Items are rated on a five-point scale ranging from 1 (strongly disagree) to 5 (strongly agree), and scores can range from 20 to 100. TAS-20 total score most often is used as continuous measure of alexithymia severity; however, cutoff scores have been established. The original TAS-20 cutoff scores are non-alexithymic, ≤ 51; intermediate, 52–60; and alexithymic, ≥ 61. Recently, Fernandes et al. (2018) published a meta-analysis exploring emotional processing impairments in obesity. The results based on 31 different studies demonstrated that individuals with obesity had higher total scores of alexithymia and higher scores on the scales measuring difficulty in identifying feelings and externally oriented thinking style, when compared with control groups. Maladaptive strategies for processing emotions, including alexithymic traits, and the tendency to counteract negative affect with comfort behaviors can partially explain the high prevalence of disordered eating behavior among patients with severe obesity.

3.3 Bariatric Data

Two recent systematic reviews have analyzed the relationship between personality traits and bariatric surgery outcomes (Bordignon et al. 2017; Generali and De Panfilis 2018). The data outlined below summarize the information reported by the two reviews and integrate it with findings from other studies.

The pre-operative personality profile of patients with better surgery outcomes is a combination of high cooperativeness, high persistence, low novelty seeking, and low impulsivity. Additional and related predictors of good outcome are an internal locus of control, a low tendency toward externalizing behaviors, a secure attachment style, and low levels of alexithymia. Such a suite of personality traits modulates a variety of individual and social behaviors that are relevant to successful pre- and post-operative treatment plans including the capacity and willingness to modify dietary habits, to increase levels of routine physical activity, to restrain alcohol consumption, and to attend monitoring appointments. This explains the strict relationship between personality profile and bariatric surgery outcomes (Fig. 3.1).

Fig. 3.1 Graphical model of the indirect relationship between personality traits and bariatric surgery outcomes. Personality traits modulate a wide range of pre- and post-operative behaviors that impact on weight loss and quality of life: TRAITS → BEHAVIORS → OUTCOMES. Legend: ↑: high, ↓: low

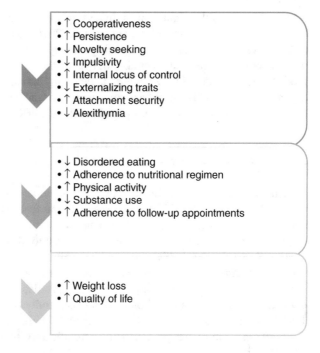

- ↑ Cooperativeness
- ↑ Persistence
- ↓ Novelty seeking
- ↓ Impulsivity
- ↑ Internal locus of control
- ↓ Externalizing traits
- ↑ Attachment security
- ↓ Alexithymia

- ↓ Disordered eating
- ↑ Adherence to nutritional regimen
- ↑ Physical activity
- ↓ Substance use
- ↑ Adherence to follow-up appointments

- ↑ Weight loss
- ↑ Quality of life

3.3.1   Temperament and Character

Individuals high on cooperativeness, who are more socially oriented, may seek and receive greater social support and thus may find it easier to adhere post-surgical diet and lifestyle changes. High persistence is associated with a greater ability to maintain a behavior for the sake of valued long-term goals. Such an ability is adaptive in the post-surgical follow-up, when individuals are required to maintain a hard-working behavior, such as attending routine diet and clinical monitoring appointments. It has been documented that the initial weight loss, together with external reinforcement (compliments, comments), is in itself highly gratifying for patients. However, these reinforcements are attenuated over time. It is likely that scoring high on persistence helps in the maintenance of the behavior acquired, as was seen in a study that indicated that, even 24 months after the surgical procedure, high persistence remains predictive of weight loss (Gordon et al. 2014). High novelty seeking is a predisposing factor for binge eating (Rotella et al. 2018) and dropping out of post-operative monitoring (Dalle Grave et al. 2018).

3.3.2   Impulsivity

Poor control of impulses promotes affect dysregulation, which may trigger pathological eating behaviors (e.g., consuming food in response to negative emotions such as depression, anxiety, or anger) and ultimately prevents patients from achieving successful weight control. In a sample of 65 patients who had undergone sleeve gastrectomy 4 years before, Schag et al. (2016) found that impulsivity had an indirect impact on weight loss through pathological eating behavior triggered by negative emotions. Kulendran et al. (2017) confirmed that poor control of impulses predicts weight reduction in patients undergoing bariatric surgery by combining psychometric (BIS-11) and behavioral measures (the *Stop Signal Reaction Time Task* and the *Temporal Discounting Task*) of impulsivity.

3.3.3   Locus of Control

Patients with an external locus of control tend to believe that they have lost control over their own diet and ability to lose weight and feel that this control cannot be regained through personal effort. Such a passive attitude is maladaptive in the post-surgical follow-up, when individuals are required to play an active role in implementing those changes to diet and lifestyle habits that are essential for a successful surgery outcome. The importance of locus of control has been shown by Perdue et al. (2018) who compared the psychological profiles of female bariatric patients divided into two groups based on their obese identity (I-obese versus I-ex-obese) 18–30 months after surgery. The participants whose obesity identity remained "I-obese" in spite of weight loss had a significantly higher external orientation toward their views of their health and weight than participants who had transitioned to see themselves as "I-ex-obese." "I-obese" individuals were oriented to see the influence of powerful others (health providers but also friends and family members) as forces instrumental in their ability to stay healthy and maintain their weight. The measures of locus of control used in this study were the MHLC and the WLOC.

3.3.4   Internalizing/Externalizing

Individual differences along the externalizing/internalizing dimension are associated with distinct problems in bariatric patients. Whereas internalizing traits seem to favor the emergence of post-operative somatic complaints and psychological distress (Bordignon et al. 2017), externalizing traits appear to be more related to less weight loss and to maladaptive eating behavior. In a sample of 498 undergoing Roux-en-Y gastric bypass, Marek et al. (2015) found that higher pre-operative scores on the scales from the Behavioral/Externalizing Dysfunction (BXD) domain of the MMPI-2-RF were associated with worse weight loss outcomes and poor adherence to follow-up. Patients scoring high scores on these scales were at greater risk for achieving suboptimal weight loss (< 50% excess weight loss) and not following up with their appointment compared with those who scored below cut-offs. Dasher et al. (2019) analyzed the impact of pre-operative personality traits as measured by the MMPI-2-RF on weight loss at 6 and 12 months post-surgery in a sample of 127 bariatric patients. At 6-month follow-up, they found a negative correlation between weight loss and the scale measuring behavioral dysregulation which reflects externalizing personality traits.

3.3.5 Attachment Style

In a sample of 108 bariatric patients, Leung et al. (2019) examined the association between attachment insecurity (as measured by the ECR-16), 2-year post-surgery disordered eating, and percent total weight loss. They found that an avoidant attachment style was a significant predictor of binge eating at 2 years post-surgery. Based on previous studies showing that avoidant attachment style predicted non-attendance at post-bariatric surgery follow-up appointments (Shakory et al. 2015) and was associated with higher rates of patient drop-out from group cognitive behavioral therapy for binge eating disorder (Tasca et al. 2011), the authors hypothesized that individuals with avoidant attachment may be non-adherent to their nutrition regimen following surgery and may not seek help, which could increase the risk of disordered eating and loss of control over eating, resulting in binge eating symptoms. In spite of its major impact on eating behavior, attachment style was not a significant predictor of percent total weight loss. Leung et al. (2019) explained such a negative finding as a possible result of the short follow-up period. In accord with such a hypothesis, another study based on a short-term (1 year after surgery) follow-up (Nancarrow et al. 2018) did not find any effect of attachment style on weight loss. In effect, the duration of the follow-up period is a critical variable for detecting the impact of pre-operative psychological variables on bariatric surgery outcomes. There is growing evidence that the findings reported during the "honeymoon" period (i.e., the first 2 years after surgery) may change substantially when re-examined 5–10 years after surgery (Galli et al. 2018).

In contrast with the negative findings reported above, Aarts et al. (2015) found that bariatric patients with higher scores on the attachment anxiety scale of the ECR were less adherent to dietary recommendations 6 months after gastric bypass surgery, influencing weight loss in a negative way during the first year after surgery. We lack long-term longitudinal studies of the association between attachment style and weight loss and other surgery outcomes. Therefore, based on available data, we should tentatively conclude that pre-operative attachment style impacts eating behavior and dietary prescriptions whereas its effect on weight loss is dubious.

3.3.6 Alexithymia

The two studies that have investigated the association between alexithymia and weight loss after bariatric surgery yielded consistent findings. Paone et al. (2019) conducted a prospective study to analyze the impact of alexithymia on bariatric surgery outcome. Seventy-five patients undergoing laparoscopic sleeve gastrectomy were enrolled. The *Toronto Alexithymia Scale* (TAS-20) was administered to patients. A postoperative weight loss check was performed at 3 and then 12 months after surgery. The TAS-20 total score was negatively correlated with the percent of excess weight loss (%EWL) at the 12-month follow-up. The analysis showed that non-alexithymic patients had a greater weight loss at 12 months after surgery compared to both probably alexithymics and alexithymic patients. Lai et al. (2019) administered the TAS-20 to 76 adult patients scheduled for bariatric surgery. At 3- and 6-month follow-up, body weight was assessed. At 6-month follow-up, alexithymic patients showed a lower percentage of total weight loss than non-alexithymic patients.

3.4   Recommendations

The assessment of personality traits is an important component of the psychosocial evaluation of bariatric patients for at least two different reasons. First, personality traits exert a major influence on a wide range of behaviors (i.e., emotion processing, adherence to post-operative lifestyle changes, attendance at follow-up appointments, eating behavior, and substance and alcohol use) that make a difference between poor and good outcomes of surgery treatment for obesity. Second, compared to psychiatric symptoms, bariatric candidates' self-report information about personality traits is less subjected to conscious alteration because personality traits are perceived as not relevant for obtaining clearance to surgery.

The findings reported in this chapter are likely to intimidate the evaluating clinician because of the number of personality traits that should be measured and the time needed to administer personality questionnaires (e.g., the MMPI-2-RF includes 338 true/false items and requires about 50 min to be completed!). Whereas this is not a problem in research studies, complexity and time are unsurmountable limits in routine clinical evaluation. Yet, these limits can be scaled down. There is a certain degree of intercorrelation among the personality traits defined by different models of personality. For example, assessing the personality traits described by the Big Five model provides an adequate picture of personality profiles and covers most of the traits reviewed in this chapter. In the Big Five model, the five dimensions of personality are openness, conscientiousness, extraversion, agreeableness, and neuroticism (mnemonic: OCEAN). The *Ten-Item Personality Inventory* (TIPI) is a brief measure of the OCEAN personality traits that requires only 5 min to be completed. Thus, if the alternative to a comprehensive battery of personality tests is just skipping personality assessment, an option like the TIPI is strongly advisable. A little is better than nothing.

KEY POINTS

Personality traits influence a wide range of behaviors that are relevant to bariatric surgery outcomes.

Compared to psychiatric symptoms, self-report of personality traits is less subjected to conscious alteration to obtain clearance to surgery.

Don't skip personality assessment! Rather, use brief questionnaires (e.g. the TIPI).

References

Aarts F, Geenen R, Gerdes VE, van de Laar A, Brandjes DP, Hinnen C. Attachment anxiety predicts poor adherence to dietary recommendations: an indirect effect on weight change 1 year after gastric bypass surgery. Obes Surg. 2015;25(4):666–72. https://doi.org/10.1007/s11695-014-1423-7.

Bordignon S, Aparício MJG, Bertoletti J, Trentini CM. Personality characteristics and bariatric surgery outcomes: a systematic review. Trends Psychiatry Psychother. 2017;39(2):124–34. Epub 2017 Jun 12. Review. https://doi.org/10.1590/2237-6089-2016-0016.

Caspi A, Moffitt TE. All for one and one for all: mental disorders in one dimension. Am J Psychiatry. 2018;175(9):831–44. Epub 2018 Apr 6. Review. PubMed PMID: 29621902; PubMed Central PMCID: PMC6120790. https://doi.org/10.1176/appi.ajp.2018.17121383.

Dalle Grave R, Calugi S, El Ghoch M. Are personality characteristics as measured by the temperament and character inventory (TCI) associated with obesity treatment outcomes? A systematic review. Curr Obes Rep. 2018;7(1):27–36. Review. https://doi.org/10.1007/s13679-018-0294-y.

Dasher NA, Sylvia A, Votruba KL. Internalizing, externalizing, and interpersonal components of the MMPI-2-RF in predicting weight change after bariatric surgery. Obes Surg. 2019;30(1):127–38. [Epub ahead of print]. https://doi.org/10.1007/s11695-019-04133-7.

Fernandes J, Ferreira-Santos F, Miller K, Torres S. Emotional processing in obesity: a systematic review and exploratory meta-analysis. Obes Rev. 2018;19(1):111–20. Epub 2017 Oct 10. Review. https://doi.org/10.1111/obr.12607.

Galli F, Cavicchioli M, Vegni E, Panizzo V, Giovanelli A, Pontiroli AE, Micheletto G. Ten years after bariatric surgery: bad quality of life promotes the need of psychological interventions. Front Psychol. 2018;9:2282. eCollection 2018. PubMed PMID: 30524346; PubMed Central PMCID: PMC6262042. https://doi.org/10.3389/fpsyg.2018.02282.

Generali I, De Panfilis C. Personality traits and weight loss surgery outcome. Curr Obes Rep. 2018;7(3):227–34. Review. https://doi.org/10.1007/s13679-018-0315-x.

Gordon PC, Sallet JA, Sallet PC. The impact of temperament and character inventory personality traits on long-term outcome of roux-en-Y gastric bypass. Obes Surg. 2014;24(10):1647–55. https://doi.org/10.1007/s11695-014-1229-7.

Kulendran M, Borovoi L, Purkayastha S, Darzi A, Vlaev I. Impulsivity predicts weight loss after obesity surgery. Surg Obes Relat Dis. 2017;13(6):1033–40. Epub 2017 Jan 4. https://doi.org/10.1016/j.soard.2016.12.031.

Lai C, Aceto P, Petrucci I, Castelnuovo G, Callari C, Giustacchini P, Sollazzi L, Mingrone G, Bellantone R, Raffaelli M. The influence of preoperative psychological factors on weight loss after bariatric surgery: a preliminary report. J Health Psychol. 2019;24(4):518–25. Epub 2016 Nov 16. https://doi.org/10.1177/1359105316677750.

Leung SE, Wnuk S, Jackson T, Cassin SE, Hawa R, Sockalingam S. Prospective study of attachment as a predictor of binge eating, emotional eating and weight loss two years after bariatric surgery. Nutrients. 2019;11(7):E1625. PubMed PMID: 31319502; PubMed Central PMCID: PMC6683092. https://doi.org/10.3390/nu11071625.

Marek RJ, Tarescavage AM, Ben-Porath YS, Ashton K, Merrell Rish J, Heinberg LJ. Using presurgical psychological testing to predict 1-year appointment adherence and weight loss in bariatric surgery patients: predictive validity and methodological considerations. Surg Obes Relat Dis. 2015;11(5):1171–81. Epub 2015 Apr 2. https://doi.org/10.1016/j.soard.2015.03.020.

Nancarrow A, Hollywood A, Ogden J, Hashemi M. The role of attachment in body weight and weight loss in bariatric patients. Obes Surg. 2018;28(2):410–4. PubMed PMID: 28681263; PubMed Central PMCID: PMC5778169. https://doi.org/10.1007/s11695-017-2796-1.

Paone E, Pierro L, Damico A, Aceto P, Campanile FC, Silecchia G, Lai C. Alexithymia and weight loss in obese patients underwent laparoscopic sleeve gastrectomy. Eat Weight Disord. 2019;24(1):129–34. Epub 2017 Mar 28. https://doi.org/10.1007/s40519-017-0381-1.

Perdue T, Schreier A, Swanson M, Neil J, Carels R. Majority of female bariatric patients retain an obese identity 18-30 months after surgery. Eat Weight Disord. 2018;25(2):357–64. [Epub ahead of print]. https://doi.org/10.1007/s40519-018-0601-3.

Rotella F, Mannucci E, Gemignani S, Lazzeretti L, Fioravanti G, Ricca V. Emotional eating and temperamental traits in eating disorders: a dimensional approach. Psychiatry Res. 2018;264:1–8. Epub 2018 Mar 23. https://doi.org/10.1016/j.psychres.2018.03.066.

Schag K, Mack I, Giel KE, Ölschläger S, Skoda EM, von Feilitzsch M, Zipfel S, Teufel M. The impact of impulsivity on weight loss four years after bariatric surgery. Nutrients. 2016;8(11):E721. PubMed PMID: 27854246; PubMed Central PMCID: PMC5133107.

Shakory S, Van Exan J, Mills JS, Sockalingam S, Keating L, Taube-Schiff M. Binge eating in bariatric surgery candidates: the role of insecure attachment and emotion regulation. Appetite. 2015;91:69–75. Epub 2015 Mar 28. https://doi.org/10.1016/j.appet.2015.03.026.

Tasca GA, Ritchie K, Balfour L. Implications of attachment theory and research for the assessment and treatment of eating disorders. Psychotherapy (Chic). 2011;48(3):249–59. Review. https://doi.org/10.1037/a0022423.

Body Image and Body Dissatisfaction

4

Abstract

Body image is the perception that individuals have of their physical self and the thoughts and feelings that result from that perception. Body dissatisfaction consists of a negative subjective evaluation of one's physical body such as figure, weight, stomach, and hips. Body dissatisfaction is greater in persons with obesity than in normal-weight persons, and compared to their respective normal-weight peers, women with obesity are more dissatisfied with their bodies than men with obesity. According to the majority of studies, body image improves after bariatric surgery. Some studies, however, showed that certain aspects of body image do not improve with weight loss or do not reach norms (e.g., average scores of people with BMIs in the normal range and no eating disorder). The rapid changes in weight and body shape following surgery are not necessarily associated with parallel changes in the way patients feel and think about their physical appearance. Thus, although a decrease of body dissatisfaction is expected after surgery, the process of rebuilding a positive body image may be lengthy and complicated. The mind–body lag is a clinical problem in which the mind retains the image of the body as obese even after massive weight loss. Bariatric patients who are not seeing themselves as they actually are after surgery and weight loss need self-direct cognitive behavioral therapy.

Keywords

Body image · Body dissatisfaction · Social stigma · Body contouring · Body image therapy

4.1   Background

Body dissatisfaction is greater in persons with obesity than in normal-weight persons, and compared to their respective normal-weight peers, women with obesity are more dissatisfied with their bodies than men with obesity (Weinberger et al. 2016). This finding explains why, especially among women, appearance concerns are a major motivation driving patients to seek surgical treatment for obesity (Libeton et al. 2004). If obesity per se is a cause of body dissatisfaction, bariatric patients may have an additional reason for showing appearance concerns. After surgery and massive weight loss, many patients report the problem of excess skin which is very troublesome.

Mental health professionals taking care of bariatric patients should pay attention to body image and body dissatisfaction because a negative body self-image is not only a source of psychological distress but also a predisposing factor for binge eating, depression, and lower self-esteem (Sharpe et al. 2018). The pathway connecting body dissatisfaction with obesity through negative affect and comfort eating has been named "the Circle of Discontent" (Marks 2015) (Fig. 4.1).

This chapter explains the concepts of body image and body dissatisfaction, provides the reader with a selective review of the psychometric instruments that can be used to measure these psychological constructs, reports data on their occurrence and correlates in bariatric patients, and offers some recommendations for their pre- and post-operative clinical management.

Fig. 4.1 The Circle of Discontent (Marks 2015). This pattern is applicable if there is a genetic predisposition for obesity or an environment in which calorically dense foods are readily available and physical activity is limited

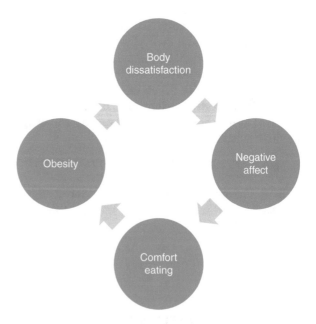

4.2   Basic Notions

Body image schemas reflect one's affect-laden beliefs about the importance and influence of appearance in one's personal life and its salience to one's self-worth and sense of self (Tylka and Wood-Barcalow 2015). Body image is the perception that individuals have of their physical self and the thoughts and feelings that result from that perception. Body image includes four distinct components. Perceptual body image is how individuals see their body. This is not always a correct representation of how the person actually looks. Affective body image is the way individuals feel about their body. This relates to the amount of satisfaction or dissatisfaction individuals feel about their shape, weight, and individual body parts. Cognitive body image is the way individuals think about their body. This can lead to preoccupation with body shape and weight. Behavioral body image encompasses those behaviors in which individuals engage as a result of their body image. When individuals are dissatisfied with the way they look, they may isolate themselves because they feel bad about their appearance or employ inappropriate behaviors as a means to change appearance.

There is evidence that body dissatisfaction, defined as negative subjective evaluations of one's physical body such as figure, weight, stomach, and hips (Stice and Shaw 2002), is not only influenced by objective anthropometric indicators (e.g., the calculation of BMI) but also built by sociocultural or psychological factors. Sociocultural factors, such as exposure to media images depicting a thin ideal, have been found to contribute to negative perceptions of one's body (Derenne and Beresin 2018). However, the impact of exposure to thin media images also appears to vary as a result of individual differences including personality traits. Negative body image is associated with higher levels of neuroticism, lower levels of extraversion, and an insecure style of attachment (Troisi et al. 2006; Allen and Walter 2016).

There are many psychometric instruments for measuring body image and body dissatisfaction in bariatric patients (Varns et al. 2018). The *Body Shape Questionnaire* (BSQ) is a self-report scale to assess body dissatisfaction caused by feelings of being fat. Psychometric evaluations of the widely used 34-item version have confirmed its retest reliability, internal consistency, construct validity, concurrent validity, discriminant validity, and its sensitivity to detect treatment-related changes. However, whether 34 items are really needed to assess a single concept has been questioned. As a consequence, several short versions of the BSQ have been developed. These derivations are the BSQ-8B, the BSQ-8C, and the BSQ-14. As for sensitivity to change, the BSQ-8C is the most favorable version of the BSQ (Pook et al. 2008). The *Multidimensional Body-Self Relations Questionnaire* (MBSRQ) is a widely used questionnaire that measures body image as a multidimensional construct. Two forms of the MBSRQ are available. The full, 69-item version consists of 10 subscales: Evaluation and Orientation vis-à-vis Appearance, Fitness, and Health/Illness, plus Overweight Preoccupation, Self-Classified Weight, and the Body Areas Satisfaction Scale (BASS). The MBSRQ-Appearance Scales (MBSRQ-AS) is a 34-item measure that consists of 5 subscales Appearance Evaluation, Appearance

Orientation, Overweight Preoccupation, Self-Classified Weight, and the BASS. The *Pictorial Body Image Assessment* (PBIA) measures the construct of perceived body size. The test consists in choosing a silhouette reflecting one's own perceived body size. The choice of a silhouette that is larger than a person's actual silhouette suggests a mind–body lag regarding body size after surgery-induced weight loss (Fig. 4.2).

4.3   Bariatric Data

One recent systematic review examined research on body image following bariatric surgery (Ivezaj and Grilo 2018). The data reported below summarize the information included in the review and integrate it with findings from other studies.

According to the majority of studies, body image improves after bariatric surgery. Some studies, however, showed that certain aspects of body image do not improve with weight loss or do not reach norms (e.g., average scores of people with BMIs in the normal range and no eating disorder). In the study by De Panfilis et al. (2007), fear of being fat, feelings of detachment from one's body, and uneasiness toward particular body parts did not improve after surgery. Six studies which reported whether post-operative body image scores were comparable to norms yielded mixed results. These findings confirm the complexity of body image schemas in severely obese patients. The social stigma experienced by patients in the time before they decide to undergo bariatric surgery builds a stable negative body image. In addition, long histories of chronic dieting and probable weight cycling can negatively and durably influence body image. The rapid changes in weight and body shape following surgery are not necessarily associated with parallel changes in the way patients feel and think about their physical appearance. Thus, although a decrease of body dissatisfaction is expected after surgery, the process of rebuilding a positive body image may be lengthy and complicated.

Patients who have undergone bariatric surgery often find they have loose, hanging skin throughout their body including the face, arms, breasts, abdomen, and thighs. These unwanted changes increase pre-existing body dissatisfaction and can cause frustration and disappointment. Body contouring following massive weight loss are procedures performed by plastic surgeons to eliminate and/or reduce excess post-bariatric surgery. Body contouring improves the shape and tone of underlying tissue and removes excess sagging fat and skin, resulting in smoother body contours and a normal appearance. Body contouring in the abdominal region is the most common procedure performed. As many as 84.5% of bariatric patients desire subsequent body contouring surgery, with greater percentages for women than men (Kitzinger et al. 2012).

Patients who undergo body contouring surgery report improvements in various body image indices compared to bariatric patients who do not undergo body contouring surgery, even after adjusting for weight loss and time since surgery. However, some patients still report high levels of body dissatisfaction following

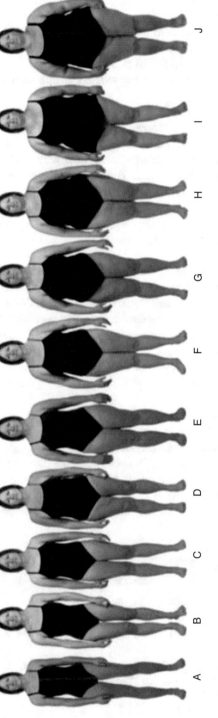

Fig. 4.2 An example of pictorial BMI-based body size guides for women. The instrument was developed to measure perception of body image. (Source: Harris C, Bradlyn A, Coffman J, et al. BMI-based body size guides for women and men: development and validation of a novel pictorial method to assess weight-related concepts. Int J Obes. 2008;32:336–42. https://doi.org/10.1038/sj.ijo.0803704), with permission

body contouring surgery. When using a body image measure like the MBSRQ that captures different body image domains, only a few body image indices improve significantly in bariatric patients who undergo body contouring surgery. Often, patients report continued dissatisfaction related to non-contoured areas. One study found that 23.5% of patients who underwent body contouring surgery sought for a second contouring surgery for another body area (Stuerz et al. 2008).

Preliminary evidence shows that there is a bidirectional relationship between pre-operative disordered eating (uncontrolled eating and binge eating) and post-operative body dissatisfaction. Patients with maladaptive eating patterns report higher levels of body dissatisfaction after bariatric surgery. However, those patients who experience an improvement of their body image after bariatric surgery report a decrease of eating pathology symptoms.

4.4   Clinical Management

Pre-operative assessment of body image provides useful information on the psychological underpinnings of negative physical self-perception that might be of value to help patients attain a more positive body image. For instance, clinicians might use this information as a method to identify potential "at risk" bariatric candidates that might benefit greatest from inclusion in body image targeted interventions. A candidate target population might be those individuals with personality traits (i.e., higher levels of neuroticism, lower levels of extraversion, and insecure attachment) that place them at greater risk of body dissatisfaction.

Post-operative follow-up should assess whether change in weight and body shape coincides with change in body image, and the personal, interpersonal, health, and lifestyle factors (e.g., physical activity) that might mediate associations between weight loss and body image. The mind–body lag is a clinical problem in which the mind retains the image of the body as obese even after massive weight loss. Bariatric patients who are not seeing themselves as they actually are after surgery and weight loss need self-direct cognitive behavioral therapy (Lewis-Smith et al. 2019).

KEY POINTS
Personality traits predict pre and post-operative body dissatisfaction.
Body image improves after bariatric surgery. Yet, rebuilding a positive body image may be lengthy and complicated.
After surgery, patients with mind-body lag need body image targeted interventions.

References

Allen MS, Walter EE. Personality and body image: a systematic review. Body Image. 2016;19:79–88. Epub 2016 Sep 14. Review. https://doi.org/10.1016/j.bodyim.2016.08.012.

De Panfilis C, Cero S, Torre M, Salvatore P, Dall'Aglio E, Adorni A, Maggini C. Changes in body image disturbance in morbidly obese patients 1 year after laparoscopic adjustable gastric banding. Obes Surg. 2007;17(6):792–9. Erratum in: Obes Surg. 2007 Jul;17(7):996.

Derenne J, Beresin E. Body image, media, and eating disorders—a 10-year update. Acad Psychiatry. 2018;42(1):129–34. Epub 2017 Oct 18. https://doi.org/10.1007/s40596-017-0832-z.

Ivezaj V, Grilo CM. The complexity of body image following bariatric surgery: a systematic review of the literature. Obes Rev. 2018;19(8):1116–40. Epub 2018 Jun 13. PubMed PMID: 29900655; PubMed Central PMCID: PMC6296375. https://doi.org/10.1111/obr.12685.

Kitzinger HB, Abayev S, Pittermann A, Karle B, Bohdjalian A, Langer FB, Prager G, Frey M. After massive weight loss: patients' expectations of body contouring surgery. Obes Surg. 2012;22(4):544–8. https://doi.org/10.1007/s11695-011-0551-6.

Lewis-Smith H, Diedrichs PC, Halliwell E. Cognitive-behavioral roots of body image therapy and prevention. Body Image. 2019;31:309–20. Epub 2019 Sep 11. Review. PubMed PMID: 31519523. https://doi.org/10.1016/j.bodyim.2019.08.009.

Libeton M, Dixon JB, Laurie C, O'Brien PE. Patient motivation for bariatric surgery: characteristics and impact on outcomes. Obes Surg. 2004;14(3):392–8.

Marks DF. Homeostatic theory of obesity. Health Psychol Open. 2015;2(1):2055102915590692. eCollection 2015 Jan. PubMed PMID: 28070357; PubMed Central PMCID: PMC5193276. https://doi.org/10.1177/2055102915590692.

Pook M, Tuschen-Caffier B, Brähler E. Evaluation and comparison of different versions of the body shape questionnaire. Psychiatry Res. 2008;158(1):67–73. Epub 2007 Nov 26.

Sharpe H, Griffiths S, Choo TH, Eisenberg ME, Mitchison D, Wall M, Neumark-Sztainer D. The relative importance of dissatisfaction, overvaluation and preoccupation with weight and shape for predicting onset of disordered eating behaviors and depressive symptoms over 15 years. Int J Eat Disord. 2018;51(10):1168–75. Epub 2018 Sep 7. PubMed PMID: 30194690; PubMed Central PMCID: PMC6289784. https://doi.org/10.1002/eat.22936.

Stice E, Shaw HE. Role of body dissatisfaction in the onset and maintenance of eating pathology: a synthesis of research findings. J Psychosom Res. 2002;53(5):985–93. Review.

Stuerz K, Piza H, Niermann K, Kinzl JF. Psychosocial impact of abdominoplasty. Obes Surg. 2008;18(1):34–8. Epub 2007 Dec 15.

Troisi A, Di Lorenzo G, Alcini S, Nanni RC, Di Pasquale C, Siracusano A. Body dissatisfaction in women with eating disorders: relationship to early separation anxiety and insecure attachment. Psychosom Med. 2006;68(3):449–53.

Tylka TL, Wood-Barcalow NL. What is and what is not positive body image? Conceptual foundations and construct definition. Body Image. 2015;14:118–29. Epub 2015 Apr 25. Review. https://doi.org/10.1016/j.bodyim.2015.04.001.

Varns JA, Fish AF, Eagon JC. Conceptualization of body image in the bariatric surgery patient. Appl Nurs Res. 2018;41:52–8. Epub 2018 Mar 26. Review. https://doi.org/10.1016/j.apnr.2018.03.008.

Weinberger NA, Kersting A, Riedel-Heller SG, Luck-Sikorski C. Body dissatisfaction in individuals with obesity compared to normal-weight individuals: a systematic review and meta-analysis. Obes Facts. 2016;9(6):424–41. Epub 2016 Dec 24. Review. PubMed PMID: 28013298; PubMed Central PMCID: PMC5644896. https://doi.org/10.1159/000454837.

Childhood Trauma

5

Abstract

Childhood trauma is a powerful risk factor for the adult onset of a variety of medical and psychiatric disorders including obesity and metabolic syndrome. Among patients seeking surgical treatment for obesity, a history of childhood trauma is relatively common and is associated with higher prevalence rates of psychiatric symptoms and mental disorders. Overall, the findings reviewed in this chapter suggest that, after surgery, bariatric patients who have been maltreated experience medical improvements and weight loss similar to those without histories of maltreatment. However, maltreated individuals often report greater levels of depression as well as mood and anxiety disorders both prior to and following surgery. Additionally, victims of childhood trauma may be at an elevated risk for psychiatric hospitalizations and suicidal behavior following surgery, especially those who are suffering from mood or substance use disorders. In patients who self-report child maltreatment and/or other early traumatic experiences on screening tests, it is essential to confirm or exclude the diagnosis of psychiatric syndromes that are known to be linked with childhood trauma, even if their symptoms do not emerge during a non-structured interview. Additionally, it is appropriate to search for the presence of those dysfunctional personality traits that are common sequelae of child maltreatment and that predict post-surgery negative outcomes.

Keywords

Early trauma · Adverse childhood experiences · Childhood maltreatment · Long-term sequelae · Ecophenotype

© Springer Nature Switzerland AG 2020
A. Troisi, *Bariatric Psychology and Psychiatry*,
https://doi.org/10.1007/978-3-030-44834-9_5

5.1   Background

In the last two decades, research and clinical studies have demonstrated that psychological traumas experienced during childhood are powerful risk factors for the onset during adulthood of a variety of medical and psychiatric disorders. Obesity is one of the possible long-term sequelae of childhood traumas (Mason et al. 2016). The Adverse Childhood Experiences Study found that severe physical, sexual, and emotional abuse in childhood were associated with 28–45% greater risks of adult obesity; moreover, 8% of obesity (BMI >30 kg/m^2) and 17% of class III obesity (BMI >40 kg/m^2) were estimated to be linked to child abuse (Williamson et al. 2002). A recent meta-analysis of 41 studies found that child maltreatment was associated with a 36% higher risk of adult obesity, with stronger association with class III obesity (Danese and Tan 2014).

The pathogenetic mechanisms linking adverse childhood experiences with adult obesity are complex and not fully understood. Early hypotheses focused exclusively on psychological and behavioral factors (e.g., anxiety and depression leading to disordered eating). More recently, emerging research has highlighted the role of childhood trauma in altering biological functions including epigenetic processes, gut microbiota, and the functionality of brain reward pathways (Mason et al. 2016; Teicher et al. 2016) (Table 5.1).

This chapter outlines basic information on childhood trauma, provides the reader with a selective review of the psychometric instruments that can be used to measure adverse childhood experiences, reports data on their occurrence and correlates in bariatric patients, and offers some recommendations for their pre- and post-operative clinical management.

Table 5.1   Possible mechanisms linking childhood trauma to adult obesity

• Diminished responsivity of dopaminergic reward circuits
• Increased levels of ghrelin
• Epigenetic changes of the PCK2 gene
• Alterations of the gut microbiome
• Depression and post-traumatic stress disorder
• Binge eating and emotional eating

5.2   Basic Notions

The WHO Consultation on Child Abuse Prevention states: *Child abuse or maltreatment constitutes all forms of physical and/or emotional ill-treatment, sexual abuse or negligent treatment or commercial or other exploitation, resulting in actual or potential harm to the child's health, survival, development or dignity in the context of a relationship of responsibility, trust or power* (World Health Organization 1999).

In research papers, the collective term "adverse childhood experiences" is often used to include all types of psychosocial stressors that negatively impact child development. In clinical settings, child maltreatment is classified into five main subtypes: physical abuse (acts of commission that cause actual physical harm or have the potential for harm), sexual abuse, emotional abuse (verbal abuse, constant criticism, intimidation), emotional neglect (failure of a caregiver to provide appropriate emotional support), and physical neglect (failure of a caregiver to provide for physical development of a child).

The overall worldwide estimated prevalence rates for self-reported maltreatment studies (mainly assessing maltreatment ever experienced during childhood) were 127/1000 for sexual abuse (76/1000 among boys and 180/1000 among girls), 226/1000 for physical abuse, 363/1000 for emotional abuse, 163/1000 for physical neglect, and 184/1000 for emotional neglect (van Ijzendoorn et al. 2019).

A variety of tools have been developed for use in adults to retrospectively assess exposure to childhood maltreatment (Saini et al. 2019). One of the most widely used instruments is the *Childhood Trauma Questionnaire* (CTQ). The CTQ is a 28-item, self-reported questionnaire administered to adults to identify traumatic childhood conditions. The CTQ includes five subscales: physical abuse, emotional abuse, sexual abuse, physical neglect, and emotional neglect. The questionnaire also includes a minimization/denial scale for detecting individuals who may be underreporting traumatic events. The scale includes 25 questions that cover items such as having emotional support, feeling loved, wearing dirty clothes, and being sexually and physically abused that tap into the five dimensions of abuse and neglect. All questions in the CTQ are preceded by "When I was growing up…" The respondent reviews the list of items and chooses the response that best describes her or his experiences. The respondent answers the questions on a five-point Likert scale: (1) never true, (2) rarely true, (3) sometimes true, (4) often true, and (5) very often true. The individual items are summed to give subscale scores from 5 to 25. The CTQ scoring manual provides guidelines for establishing thresholds for four levels of abuse/neglect for each subscale: none; moderate; severe; extreme.

Another important and simpler metric is the *Adverse Childhood Experience* (ACE) score, which emphasizes multiplicity of exposure rather than severity. Three categories of childhood abuse are assessed: emotional, physical, or contact sexual abuse, along with five categories of household dysfunction: exposure to substance abuse, mental illness, violent treatment of mother or stepmother, incarceration for criminal behavior, and parental separation, divorce, or death. Subjects are defined as exposed to a category if they responded "yes" to one or more of the questions in that category. The number of categories reported (range 0–8) are summed to produce the

ACE score. This turned out to be a simple, but highly effective strategy, yielding a multiplicity score that seems to capture the extent of exposure to childhood adversity. The most recent version of the ACE score (Wave II) added two categories: physical and emotional neglect.

A limitation of all instruments (including the CTQ and the ACE) used in adults to retrospectively assess exposure to childhood maltreatment is that none collects detailed information on how exposure levels changed across development. This information is of fundamental importance as there may be sensitive periods when experience exerts maximal effects on the developmental trajectory of specific brain regions and risk for psychopathology. To overcome this methodological limitation, Teicher and Parigger (2015) developed the *Maltreatment and Abuse Chronology of Exposure* (MACE) scale to gauge the severity of exposure to ten types of maltreatment (emotional neglect, non-verbal emotional abuse, parental physical maltreatment, parental verbal abuse, peer emotional abuse, peer physical bullying, physical neglect, sexual abuse, witnessing violence between parents, and witnessing violence to siblings) during each year of childhood. The MACE provides an overall severity score and multiplicity score (the number of types of maltreatment experienced).

5.3   Bariatric Data

Among patients seeking surgical treatment for obesity, a history of childhood trauma is relatively common and is associated with higher prevalence rates of mental disorders and psychiatric symptoms.

Among 340 bariatric candidates, Grilo et al. (2005) found that 69% of patients self-reported childhood maltreatment: 46% reported emotional abuse, 29% reported physical abuse, 32% reported sexual abuse, 49% reported emotional neglect, and 32% reported physical neglect. Except for higher rates of emotional abuse reported by women, different forms of maltreatment did not differ significantly by sex. Different forms of maltreatment were generally not associated with binge eating, current BMI, or eating disorder features. However, emotional abuse was associated with higher eating concerns and body dissatisfaction, and emotional neglect was associated with higher eating concerns. In terms of psychological functioning, emotional abuse and emotional neglect were associated with higher depression and lower self-esteem, and physical abuse was associated with higher depression.

Wildes et al. (2008) reported that, in a sample of 260 bariatric candidates, approximately 66% of participants had a history of childhood maltreatment. Individuals reporting childhood maltreatment had a greater number of lifetime DSM-IV Axis I diagnoses than did those without, although the effect for physical neglect was no longer significant after controlling for multiple comparisons. With respect to specific Axis I diagnoses, a history of emotional or sexual abuse was associated with increased rates of lifetime mood and anxiety disorder diagnoses. Emotional neglect also was associated with increased rates of mood disorder diagnoses, and physical abuse was associated with increased rates of substance use disorders. In a sample of 368 bariatric patients, Orcutt et al. (2019) found that 66.6% of females and 47.0% of males reported at least one form of childhood trauma. Among women, the presence and greater severity of emotional or physical abuse or neglect was associated with a higher risk of history of psychopathology (i.e., major depressive disorder, post-traumatic stress disorder, other anxiety disorder, alcohol use disorder, and binge eating disorder), suicidal ideation/behavior, and antidepressant use. These associations were independent of age, race, education, body mass index, and childhood sexual abuse. Childhood sexual abuse was independently associated with a history of suicidal ideation/behavior and antidepressant use only.

Some studies have investigated the impact of childhood trauma on short- and long-term outcomes of bariatric surgery. Grilo et al. (2006) investigated the prognostic significance of childhood maltreatment in 137 extremely obese patients undergoing gastric bypass surgery who completed a questionnaire battery before surgery and again 12 months after surgery. Significant and clinically robust improvements in weight and in all measures of eating and psychological functioning were observed at 12 months after surgery. Patients who reported histories of childhood sexual abuse and other forms of childhood maltreatment differed little from patients who reported no childhood maltreatment in body mass index, eating disorder features, and psychological functioning both pre- and post-operatively at 12-month follow-up. Patients who reported childhood sexual abuse had statistically significantly higher levels of depression at 12 months after surgery, although the depression levels represented significant reductions from pre-surgery and fell within the non-depressed range. Another short-term study was recently published by Peterhänsel et al. (2019) who focused on the association between childhood maltreatment and outcomes 6 and 12 months after a bariatric procedure in 120 patients. Childhood maltreatment did not impact the course of body weight, depression, and eating disorder pathology from pre- to post-surgery.

As for other post-surgery outcomes, findings from long-term studies are different from those reported by short-term studies (i.e., within 2 years after surgery). King et al. (2019) conducted a 7-year longitudinal study to examine associations between childhood trauma and changes in depressive symptoms, eating pathology, and weight in 96 bariatric patients who had undergone Roux-en-Y Gastric Bypass (RYGB). Childhood emotional abuse, emotional neglect, and physical neglect, but not sexual abuse or physical abuse, were significantly associated with less improvement or worsening depressive and eating pathology symptoms. All types of maltreatment were associated with less improvement or worsening in eating concern and shape concern scores. By contrast, there was no significant association between childhood maltreatment and weight loss or regain. The authors concluded that, although childhood trauma did not affect weight outcomes after RYGB, those who experienced childhood trauma had less improvement in depressive symptomology and eating pathology and therefore might benefit from clinical intervention.

One study that reported a negative association between childhood maltreatment and post-surgery weight loss was published by Lodhia et al. (2015) who enrolled a sample of 223 patients undergoing RYGB, sleeve gastrectomy, or adjustable gastric band. Compared to participants with no history of childhood trauma, patients with a history of childhood abuse, neglect, and household dysfunction had a higher post-operative BMI at 6 months and 12 months post-operatively. Notably, this was a study with a short follow-up period.

Overall, the findings reviewed in this section suggest that bariatric surgery patients who have been maltreated experience medical improvements and weight loss similar to those without histories of maltreatment. However, maltreated individuals often report greater levels of depression as well as mood and anxiety disorders both prior to and following surgery. Additionally, victims of childhood trauma may be at an elevated risk for psychiatric hospitalizations and suicidal behavior following surgery, especially those who are suffering from mood or substance use disorders (Mitchell et al. 2013). An important caveat is that methodological differences between studies (e.g., different measures of childhood trauma, variable length of follow-up period, different measures of outcome) make the comparison between their findings difficult.

5.4   Clinical Management

Pre-operative investigation of childhood trauma is clinically important for two reasons. First, patients with adverse early experiences have an increased likelihood of being diagnosed with a wide range of psychiatric disorders that may impact bariatric surgery outcomes. In patients who self-report child maltreatment and/or other early traumatic experiences on screening tests, it is essential to confirm or exclude the diagnosis of psychiatric syndromes that are known to be linked with childhood trauma, even if their symptoms do not emerge during a non-structured interview (e.g., a patient who does not mention the typical symptoms of borderline personality disorder). Additionally, even if the patient does not fulfill the diagnostic criteria for a psychiatric disorder, it is appropriate to search for the presence of those dysfunctional personality traits that are common sequelae of child maltreatment and that predict post-surgery negative outcomes (e.g., insecure attachment, disturbed body image, alexithymia).

The second reason is probably more important although its clinical applicability is currently limited. Phenotypic expression of psychopathology is strongly influenced by exposure to maltreatment, leading to a constellation of "ecophenotypes" (Teicher and Samson 2013). Maltreated individuals with depressive, anxiety, and substance use disorders show an earlier age of onset, greater symptom severity, more comorbidity, increased risk for suicide, and poorer treatment response than non-maltreated individuals with the same diagnoses. While these ecophenotypes fit within conventional diagnostic boundaries, they likely represent distinct subtypes. Recognition of this distinction may be useful in predicting the post-surgery outcomes of bariatric patients. Pre- and post-operative treatment guidelines and algorithms may be enhanced if maltreated and non-maltreated patients with the same diagnostic labels (e.g., disordered eating and depression) are differentiated.

Key points
Among patients seeking surgical treatment for obesity, a history of childhood trauma is relatively common.
Maltreated individuals often report greater levels of depression as well as mood and anxiety disorders both prior to and following surgery.
Victims of childhood trauma may be at an elevated risk for psychiatric hospitalizations and suicidal behavior following surgery
In high-risk patients, prevention of post-surgery psychiatric complications requires focused intervention.

References

Danese A, Tan M. Childhood maltreatment and obesity: systematic review and meta-analysis. Mol Psychiatry. 2014;19(5):544–54. Epub 2013 May 21. Review. https://doi.org/10.1038/mp.2013.54.

Grilo CM, Masheb RM, Brody M, Toth C, Burke-Martindale CH, Rothschild BS. Childhood maltreatment in extremely obese male and female bariatric surgery candidates. Obes Res. 2005;13(1):123–30.

Grilo CM, White MA, Masheb RM, Rothschild BS, Burke-Martindale CH. Relation of childhood sexual abuse and other forms of maltreatment to 12-month postoperative outcomes in extremely obese gastric bypass patients. Obes Surg. 2006;16(4):454–60.

King WC, Hinerman A, Kalarchian MA, Devlin MJ, Marcus MD, Mitchell JE. The impact of childhood trauma on change in depressive symptoms, eating pathology, and weight after Roux-en-Y gastric bypass. Surg Obes Relat Dis. 2019;15(7):1080–8. Epub 2019 Apr 17. PubMed PMID: 31153892; PubMed Central PMCID: PMC6702081. https://doi.org/10.1016/j.soard.2019.04.012.

Lodhia NA, Rosas US, Moore M, Glaseroff A, Azagury D, Rivas H, Morton JM. Do adverse childhood experiences affect surgical weight loss outcomes? J Gastrointest Surg. 2015;19(6):993–8. Epub 2015 Apr 2. https://doi.org/10.1007/s11605-015-2810-7.

Mason SM, Bryn Austin S, Bakalar JL, Boynton-Jarrett R, Field AE, Gooding HC, Holsen LM, Jackson B, Neumark-Sztainer D, Sanchez M, Sogg S, Tanofsky-Kraff M, Rich-Edwards JW. Child maltreatment's heavy toll: the need for trauma-informed obesity prevention. Am J Prev Med. 2016;50(5):646–9. Epub 2015 Dec 11. PubMed PMID: 26689978; PubMed Central PMCID: PMC4905569. https://doi.org/10.1016/j.amepre.2015.11.004.

Mitchell JE, Crosby R, de Zwaan M, Engel S, Roerig J, Steffen K, Gordon KH, Karr T, Lavender J, Wonderlich S. Possible risk factors for increased suicide following bariatric surgery. Obesity (Silver Spring). 2013;21(4):665–72. Review. PubMed PMID: 23404774; PubMed Central PMCID: PMC4372842. https://doi.org/10.1002/oby.20066.

Orcutt M, King WC, Kalarchian MA, Devlin MJ, Marcus MD, Garcia L, Steffen KJ, Mitchell JE. The relationship between childhood maltreatment and psychopathology in adults undergoing bariatric surgery. Surg Obes Relat Dis. 2019;15(2):295–303. Epub 2018 Nov 15.

PubMed PMID: 31010652; PubMed Central PMCID: PMC6481306. https://doi.org/10.1016/j. soard.2018.11.009.

Peterhänsel C, Nagl M, Wagner B, Dietrich A, Kersting A. Childhood maltreatment in bariatric patients and its association with postoperative weight, depressive, and eating disorder symptoms. Eat Weight Disord. 2019. [Epub ahead of print]. https://doi.org/10.1007/s40519-019-00720-w.

Saini SM, Hoffmann CR, Pantelis C, Everall IP, Bousman CA. Systematic review and critical appraisal of child abuse measurement instruments. Psychiatry Res. 2019;272:106–13. Epub 2018 Dec 13. https://doi.org/10.1016/j.psychres.2018.12.068.

Teicher MH, Parigger A. The 'Maltreatment and Abuse Chronology of Exposure' (MACE) scale for the retrospective assessment of abuse and neglect during development. PLoS One. 2015;10(2):e0117423. eCollection 2015. PubMed PMID: 25714856; PubMed Central PMCID: PMC4340880. https://doi.org/10.1371/journal.pone.0117423.

Teicher MH, Samson JA. Childhood maltreatment and psychopathology: a case for ecophenotypic variants as clinically and neurobiologically distinct subtypes. Am J Psychiatry. 2013;170(10):1114–33. Review. PubMed PMID: 23982148; PubMed Central PMCID: PMC3928064. https://doi.org/10.1176/appi.ajp.2013.12070957.

Teicher MH, Samson JA, Anderson CM, Ohashi K. The effects of childhood maltreatment on brain structure, function and connectivity. Nat Rev Neurosci. 2016;17(10):652–66. Review. https://doi.org/10.1038/nrn.2016.111.

van Ijzendoorn MH, Bakermans-Kranenburg MJ, Coughlan B, Reijman S. Annual research review: umbrella synthesis of meta-analyses on child maltreatment antecedents and interventions: differential susceptibility perspective on risk and resilience. J Child Psychol Psychiatry. 2019. [Epub ahead of print] Review. https://doi.org/10.1111/jcpp.13147.

Wildes JE, Kalarchian MA, Marcus MD, Levine MD, Courcoulas AP. Childhood maltreatment and psychiatric morbidity in bariatric surgery candidates. Obes Surg. 2008;18(3):306–13. Epub 2008 Jan 12. PubMed PMID: 18193182; PubMed Central PMCID: PMC2893145. https://doi.org/10.1007/s11695-007-9292-y.

Williamson DF, Thompson TJ, Anda RF, Dietz WH, Felitti V. Body weight and obesity in adults and self-reported abuse in childhood. Int J Obes Relat Metab Disord. 2002;26(8):1075–82.

World Health Organization Consultation on Child Abuse Prevention. Violence and Injury Prevention Team & Global Forum for Health Research. Report of the consultation on child abuse prevention, 29-31 March 1999, WHO. Geneva: World Health Organization; 1999.

Eating Disorders

6

Abstract

Eating disorders are probably the area of psychopathology most relevant to bariatric surgery. Obese patients seeking bariatric surgery have a high prevalence of eating disordered behavior, and binge eating disorder is frequently diagnosed in bariatric candidates. A small, but significant, number of bariatric patients develop eating disorders after surgery. Pre-surgery assessment should investigate past and/or current symptoms of both major eating disorders (i.e., anorexia nervosa, bulimia nervosa, and binge eating disorder) and other maladaptive eating patterns that are common in bariatric patients (i.e., grazing, night eating syndrome, emotional eating, loss-of-control eating, and food addiction). Until recently, a pre-operative diagnosis of eating disorder was considered a major contraindication to bariatric surgery. This limitation has been reduced over time and bariatric surgery interventions can now be suitable for selected patients with current eating disorders, even if clinical outcomes and the extent of weight loss depend on the persistence or re-emergence of eating pathology after the intervention.

Keywords

Binge eating disorder · Bulimia · Anorexia · Grazing, Night eating syndrome, Emotional eating, Loss-of-control eating · Food addiction

6.1 Background

According to DSM-5, feeding and eating disorders are characterized by a persistent disturbance of eating or eating-related behavior that results in the altered consumption or absorption of food and that significantly impairs physical health or psychosocial functioning. The three major eating disorders listed in the DSM-5 are anorexia nervosa, bulimia nervosa, and binge eating disorder.

© Springer Nature Switzerland AG 2020

A. Troisi, *Bariatric Psychology and Psychiatry*,

https://doi.org/10.1007/978-3-030-44834-9_6

Eating disorders are probably the area of psychopathology most relevant to bariatric surgery. Obese patients seeking bariatric surgery have a high prevalence of eating disordered behavior, and binge eating disorder is frequently diagnosed in bariatric candidates. A small, but significant, number of bariatric patients develop eating disorders after surgery. Finally, pre- and post-operative eating disordered behaviors can impact on bariatric surgery outcomes.

This chapter illustrates assessment procedures for diagnosing eating disorders, outlines basic notions on their prevalence and treatment, and reviews published data on the indications, contraindications, and outcomes of bariatric surgery in patients with eating disorders (analyzed in order of their relevance to bariatric surgery). In addition to the three major eating disorders listed in the DSM-5 (i.e., anorexia nervosa, bulimia nervosa, and binge eating disorder), the chapter deals with other abnormal eating patterns that are common in bariatric patients (i.e., grazing, night eating syndrome, emotional eating, loss-of-control eating, and food addiction) and that should be detected throughout both pre- and post-operative psychosocial assessment (Table 6.1).

6.2   Assessment

Clinical interview schedules are the gold standard method for the diagnosis of eating disorders. However, their routine application is not always feasible as they are laborious and must be performed by trained mental health professionals. Therefore, self-report questionnaires are preferred as screening tools for the assessment of eating pathology in busy routine clinical conditions. Ideally, a good screening instrument should be highly sensitive in order to identify the majority of affected patients with eating disorders. On the other hand, its specificity is less relevant, since the diagnosis of eating disorders needs to be confirmed in any case by clinical interview.

Parker and Brennan (2015) published a systematic review of the literature in order to select the most appropriate assessment measures of eating pathology in bariatric surgery candidates. Among the interviews currently available, they recommend the *Eating Disorder Examination* (EDE). The EDE is a semi-structured interview conducted by a trained clinician to assess the psychopathology associated with the diagnosis of an eating disorder. The EDE is rated through the use of four subscales and a global score. The four subscales are: (1) restraint; (2) food concern; (3) shape concern; and (4) weight concern. The questions concern the frequency in which the patient engages in behaviors indicative of an eating disorder over a 28-day period. The test is scored on a 7-point scale from 0 to 6 with a zero score indicating not having engaged in the questioned behavior.

Table 6.1   Eating disorders and maladaptive eating patterns in bariatric patients

DIAGNOSIS	PRE-SURGERY	POST-SURGERY
Binge eating disorder (BED)	High prevalence. Mixed findings as a negative predictor of outcome	Objective binge eating may be replaced by subjective binge eating or grazing
Bulimia nervosa	Prevalence low, probably because of patients' underreporting	Associated with medical complications
Anorexia nervosa	Sometimes present in patients' past history	May develop de novo after surgery
Grazing	High prevalence	Mixed findings. May be a negative predictor of weight loss
Night eating syndrome	Uncertain prevalence (8–55%)	No impact on weight loss. Improves after surgery
Emotional eating	Associated with negative affectivity	No impact on weight loss
Loss-of-control eating	Overlapping with BED	Negative predictor of weight loss
Food addiction	High prevalence. Associated with broad psychopathology	Improves up to 12 months after surgery

Among the self-rated questionnaires, they recommend the *Binge Eating Scale* (BES). The BES includes 16 items; a global score for eating disturbance is obtained by summing the responses to the 16 items. As a screen for binge eating, the BES demonstrates good sensitivity (94%) and has a two-factor construct model (feelings/cognitions and behaviors) that is confirmed for people seeking bariatric surgery. These factor scores could be beneficial when designing treatment plans including cognitive behavioral therapy. The BES also demonstrates good reliability (IC $\alpha = 0.87$) and benefits from straightforward scoring and interpretability with a validated cut score of ≥ 17 (Barclay et al. 2015).

When selecting the assessment tools to use in bariatric patients, mental health professionals have a wide choice of measures and they can rely on comprehensive reviews that are helpful to take an informed decision (Parker and Brennan 2015; Barclay et al. 2015; Marek et al. 2016; Parker et al. 2016). What is important is to make the choice on the basis of specific criteria that should be weighed against the context where the assessment takes place (Table 6.2).

Table 6.2 Criteria for selecting measures of eating pathology

CRITERION	RATIONALE
Patient burden	Is the length and content of the measure acceptable to patients given the context where the assessment takes place?
Reliability	Is the test-retest reproducibility good enough?
Validity	Does the measure target the dimensions of eating pathology that are under investigation?
Sensitivity	Is the measure a good screening test? Is the measure able to identify those patients who need a structured interview?
Clinician burden	How easy is the measure to administer and score? Are the results straightforward to interpret?

ASSESSMENT TIPS
Diagnostic investigation should target the entire spectrum of eating pathology.
Positive screening tests should be followed by structured interview.
Patients may hide information that could make them not eligible for bariatric surgery.
Post-surgery assessment is as much important as pre-operative diagnostic evaluation.

6.3   Binge Eating Disorder

Binge eating disorder (BED) is the most common eating disorder. DSM-5 diagnostic criteria require the presence of recurrent episodes of eating significantly more food in a short period of time than most people would eat under similar circumstances, with episodes marked by feelings of lack of control. Someone with binge eating disorder may eat too quickly, even when he or she is not hungry. The person may have feelings of guilt, embarrassment, or disgust and may binge eat alone to hide the behavior. This disorder is associated with marked distress and occurs, on average, at least once a week over 3 months. Unlike bulimia nervosa, binge eating episodes are not followed by compensatory behaviors and this typically leads to obesity. BED is more common in women than men and in obese individuals (5% to 30%), especially those who are severely obese and those seeking obesity treatment. It typically emerges in early adulthood and may persist well beyond midlife

(Brownley et al. 2016). The gender difference in prevalence rates observed in the general population is minimal or absent in bariatric patients.

Psychotherapies are the most validated interventions for BED and should be considered as first-line treatments. Cognitive-behavioral therapy (CBT) is widely used in both individual and group settings. Alternative and effective psychotherapies are the dialectic-behavioral therapy (DBT) and interpersonal therapy (IPT), with this latter technique focusing on personal relations and role transitions that could have a predisposing and maintaining role in BED (Amianto et al. 2015).

Antidepressants, especially selective serotonin reuptake inhibitors (SSRI) at high doses, are the most widely used medications in BED treatment, showing efficacy on eating impulsiveness but also on anxiety and depressive symptoms, with supposed secondary positive effects on emotional eating due to lowering of negative affect that trigger binges. Recently, the indications for lisdexamfetamine (LDX), a central nervous system stimulant, were expanded to include treatment of moderate to severe BED (Ward and Citrome 2018). In clinical trials, LDX demonstrated statistical and clinical superiority over placebo in reducing binge eating days per week at doses of 50 and 70 mg daily. Commonly reported side effects of LDX include dry mouth, insomnia, weight loss, and headache; and its use should be avoided in patients with known structural cardiac abnormalities, cardiomyopathy, serious heart arrhythmia, or coronary artery disease. As with all CNS stimulants, the risk of abuse needs to be assessed prior to prescribing.

6.3.1   Bariatric Data

The relationship between BED and bariatric surgery has been recently reviewed by Tess et al. (2019). The prevalence rates of BED in bariatric candidates vary widely because of major differences in diagnostic instruments (structured interviews vs. self-report questionnaires) and inclusion/exclusion criteria. In the 21 studies analyzed by the review, prevalence ranged from 2% to 53%. In patients seeking bariatric surgery, BED is associated with an increased prevalence of comorbid psychiatric disorders, especially mood disorders (Jones-Corneille et al. 2012).

Despite the great number of studies focusing on pre-surgery eating disorders, no consensus has been reached on the association between pre-operative BED and weight loss outcomes after surgery. There are studies showing that patients with and without BED show similar outcomes in terms of after-surgery weight loss and weight regain (e.g., Busetto et al. 2005; Alger-Mayer et al. 2009). However, other studies failed to confirm that BED is not a negative predictor of outcome. One variable that can explain mixed findings is the presence after the surgery of symptoms resembling BED. Ivezaj et al. (2018) have described the "Bariatric Binge-Eating Disorder" (Bar-BED) defined as an eating pathology meeting all criteria for DSM-5 BED, except for the requirement of an unusually large amount of food. They found that, after sleeve gastrectomy surgery, bariatric outcomes were worse in patients with such a diagnosis. Thus, it is likely that a negative impact of BED on bariatric outcomes is exclusive to, or more frequent in, those patients who retain their pre-surgery eating pathology (Niego et al. 2007). Morseth et al. (2016) conducted a 5-year follow-up study in order to compare the impact of different surgical procedures on self-reported eating disorder symptoms. Before surgery, the prevalence of binge eating was 29% in the Roux-en-Y gastric bypass (RYGB) group and 32% in the biliopancreatic diversion with duodenal switch (DS) group. The prevalence improved during the first 12 months after surgery in both groups. After 5 years, the prevalence of binge eating episodes was 22% in the RYGB group and 7% in the DS group. The difference between groups throughout follow-up was non-significant.

6.4   Bulimia Nervosa

Bulimia nervosa is characterized by frequent episodes of uncontrolled binge eating followed by inappropriate compensatory behaviors to avoid weight gain. When patients with bulimia nervosa binge due to strong food cravings, they tend to feel guilty and as a result undergo compensatory weight loss behaviors such as vomiting, using laxatives, exercising excessively, and alternating with periods of starvation. Bulimia nervosa is much more prevalent in young women. The estimated prevalence in women aged 15–40 is 1–2%. Comorbidity with other psychiatric disorders is relatively high, especially with depression, anxiety, deliberate self-harm, substance misuse, and borderline personality disorder.

Treatment strategies are widely overlapping with those applied in BED. A form of cognitive-behavioral therapy specifically adapted for bulimia nervosa (CBT-BN) can be combined with psychoeducation about nutrition. Useful behavioral techniques include food diary to monitor eating/purging patterns, planned small and regular meals, and eating in company. Fluoxetine at high dose (60 mg/day) is the SSRI of choice. Inpatient treatment is required for cases of suicide risk and severe electrolyte imbalance. Approximately 50% of patients with bulimia nervosa make a complete recovery.

6.4.1   Bariatric Data

Data on bulimia nervosa in bariatric patients are scarce. During pre-operative screening, patients are likely to be guarded about diagnostic information they are willing to share with mental health professionals. This is typically caused by the fact that they are fearful that the information they provide may exclude them from being eligible for surgery. The discrepancy between self-reported prevalence of BED and bulimia nervosa among patients seeking bariatric surgery is strikingly large. For example, in a small study of 60 bariatric patients, Morseth et al. (2016) found that 30% of the participants reported "objective bulimic episodes" before surgery. Yet, the authors' definition of bulimic episodes (eating an unusually large amount of food with a sense of having lost control over eating) did not include compensatory behaviors which are the diagnostic core of bulimia nervosa. Thus, the prevalence they found should be better understood as reflecting binge eating. Only two participants reported self-induced vomiting. de Zwaan et al. (2010) reported that only two of the 59 participants in their study met criteria for bulimia nervosa prior to surgery. Both of these patients had a poor outcome.

Although there is no general consensus if bulimia nervosa should be considered an absolute contraindication to bariatric surgery, there is evidence that patients combining binge eating and purging behaviors are at risk for medical complications after surgery (Sekuła et al. 2019). Water and electrolyte imbalance, acid and alkaline imbalance, and esophageal injuries are especially dangerous in the postoperative period in patients in whom bulimia has not been treated before bariatric surgery. Esophageal injuries, if present for a longer period, may lead to erosions, dangerous bleeding or even esophageal rupture. Deficiencies associated with surgery alone, such as deficiencies of vitamins, minerals or protein may progress due to the chronic use of laxatives, dehydrating agents, and self-induced vomiting. Since gastroesophageal reflux disease is often observed in obese patients and its symptoms may also accompany bulimia nervosa, such patients have to be carefully monitored. It is well known that chronic esophageal reflux may favor the development of Barrett's esophagus, which is a precancerous condition involving intestinal metaplasia of the esophageal epithelium.

A further indication of the uncertainty in this area of bariatric psychiatry is the study of Yashkov and Bekuzarov (2006). Six young women with pre-operative bulimia nervosa underwent biliopancreatic diversion (BPD). According to the authors: *All 6 patients were cured or significantly improved of bulimic symptoms soon after BPD. Weight loss was very good and never reached an undesirably low level. Patient satisfaction was high.* The interesting aspect of this study was that patients' BMIs were lower than the threshold indicated by guidelines as an indication for bariatric surgery. Thus, bariatric surgery was chosen as a treatment for bulimia nervosa, even though the authors cautiously stated: *We do not consider that every patient suffering from bulimia nervosa should be a potential candidate for BPD.* (p. 1437).

6.5 Anorexia Nervosa

By definition, bariatric patients are obese. Thus, anorexia nervosa is expected to have no relevance to psychosocial evaluation of patients assessed before surgery and throughout the follow-up period after surgery. This is not the case for two different reasons. First, some obese patients seeking bariatric surgery may have experienced symptoms of anorexia nervosa in the past. A personal history of anorexia nervosa is likely to reflect an abnormal attitude toward eating and weight control that may be reinforced in the post-operative period (Shear and DeFilippis 2015). Second, some bariatric patients develop pathological patterns of restrictive caloric intake after surgery. For these reasons, mental health professionals who take care of bariatric patients should evaluate past and current symptoms related to anorexia nervosa.

Patients with anorexia nervosa restrict what they eat and may compulsively overexercise to maintain an excessively low body weight. The DSM-5 diagnosis requires the presence of: (1) BMI < 17.5; (2) morbid fear of fatness; (3) deliberate weight loss; (4) distorted body image. Anorexia nervosa usually begins in mid-adolescence and is much more prevalent in young women than in any other age/gender class. There are two different diagnostic subtypes: "restricting type" with minimal food intake and strenuous exercise, and "binge-eating/purging type" with episodic binge eating and compensatory behaviors such as self-induced vomiting and laxative use.

Treatment failure is relatively common in patients with anorexia nervosa, especially in cases with high frequency of purging and/or late onset. For adolescents, family interventions are first line. For adults, effective psychological therapies include CBT and IPT. Antidepressants and atypical antipsychotics are of little utility. Hospitalization is required when BMI is lower than 14 and in patients with suicide risk or severe physical sequelae of starvation or purging.

6.5.1 Bariatric Data

Published reports of anorexia nervosa in bariatric patients are exclusively case histories. This is understandable considering the rarity of anorexia nervosa in obese patients seeking surgical treatment. For example, in a series of 2800 patients who underwent gastroplasty or gastric bypass, Deitel (2002) encountered only two patients who slowly slipped into intractable anorexia nervosa after surgery. Most case reports refer to patients with pre-surgery histories of eating disorders characterized by impulsiveness and feeding disinhibition (Conceição et al. 2013). However, in some cases, the patient denied the presence of past or current symptoms of abnormal eating behavior (Tortorella et al. 2015) or developed severe anorexia associated with abnormal plasma levels of gut hormones (Pucci et al. 2015). It is likely that different pathogenic pathways can lead to post-surgery anorexia nervosa.

Another unsolved question is if post-surgery anorexia nervosa is a syndrome fully overlapping with that described by DSM-5 or if instead it is best classified as a distinct eating disorder. Favoring the latter option, Segal et al. (2004) have suggested a specific set of criteria for the "post-surgical eating avoidance disorder." The syndrome is characterized by: (1) previous history of morbid obesity, followed by bariatric surgery within the past 2 years; (2) the use of purgative strategies or excessive reduction of food intake; and (3) rapid weight loss.

6.6 Maladaptive Eating Patterns

In addition to anorexia nervosa, bulimia nervosa, and binge eating disorder, there are other conditions that reflect abnormal eating patterns associated with psychological dysfunction. These conditions should be assessed during pre- and postoperative psychosocial evaluation because they can impact bariatric surgery outcomes. It is worth noting that the abnormal eating patterns described below are defined and discussed as distinct conditions by research and clinical studies. However, there is a high degree of overlapping among them and the major eating disorders classified by the DSM-5.

6.6.1   Grazing

Grazing is defined as the unstructured, repetitive eating of small amounts of food over a longer time period, outside of planned meals, and snacks and/or not in response to hunger or satiety sensations (Conceição et al. 2014). Other terms that have been used to indicate this abnormal eating pattern are "constant overeating," "picking and nibbling," and "chaotic/unstructured eating." Grazing differs from snacking which is an eating episode in which the amount is known at the outset with some certainty and which lacks a repetitious element. Grazing also differs from subjective binge eating which always entails a sense of loss of control and where the amount consumed is considered large by those engaging in this behavior. However, it is worth noting that some studies considered grazing to include a degree of loss of control over eating, while others explicitly excluded loss of control from their definition of grazing.

Pre-surgery prevalence of grazing among bariatric candidates is around 30%. There are specific instruments for assessing grazing including the *Grazing Questionnaire* and the *Repetitive Eating Questionnaire* (Rep(eat)-Q). Questions focusing on grazing are also included in the investigator-based interview *Eating Disorders Examination-Bariatric Surgery Version* (EDE-BSV).

Heriseanu et al. (2017) have recently published a comprehensive review on the relationship between grazing, obesity, and eating disorders. The data from bariatric patients included in the review are reported below. Data on pre-operative grazing as a predictor of outcome are not consistent. Busetto et al. (2002) found that pre-operative grazing did not predict successful post-surgery weight loss (defined as the percentage of excess weight loss, %EWL > 50), post-surgical weight loss failure (%EWL < 20), or weight regain (> 10% EWL) 1–3 years after surgery. Burgmer et al. (2005) found no significant difference in average weight loss at 12-month post-bariatric surgery follow-up between patients with and without baseline grazing. Unlike the studies above, Colles et al. (2008) found that patients with pre-surgical grazing had lost less weight compared to those without grazing after controlling for BMI and that a majority (94.1%) continued to graze. Poole et al. (2005) found that patients with baseline grazing were more likely to display poor post-surgical compliance with follow-ups/dietary advice.

Also the data on post-operative grazing are not consistent. At the 12-month post-surgery follow-up by Colles et al. (2008), patients with post-surgical grazing had lost less weight than those without grazing. In addition, over 60% of baseline participants with BED reported post-operative grazing. This finding supports the observation that patients who binge eat pre-surgery convert to a grazing pattern post-surgery, once binge episodes are no longer physically possible (Saunders 2004). Those who grazed also reported a higher number of gastrointestinal symptoms. de Zwaan et al. (2010) did not find an association between grazing 1.9 years post-operatively and the amount of postoperative weight loss. Conceição et al. (2014) reported mixed effects: grazing at 6–24 months' follow-up was not significantly associated with weight loss; however, there was a significant association with weight regain. De Cesare et al. (2014) did not find a significant difference in the number of participants with grazing among those with adequate and inadequate weight loss at 2–3 years after surgery. However, the number of patients was small: 0/18 vs. 2/12 participants grazed, respectively.

In the longer term, Kofman et al. (2010) reported that grazing at 3–10 years of follow-up (mean = 4.2 years) was positively correlated with weight regain and negatively correlated with EWL. In this study, participants who reported grazing two or more times a week had greater weight regain and less EWL than those with less frequent grazing. Mack et al. (2016) reported that at 1.75–6.67 years of follow-up (mean = 4.0 years), patients who grazed had lower %EWL (42.1 vs. 55.3) and higher BMIs (40.4 vs. 35.5), compared to those who did not graze. Similarly, Nicolau et al. (2015) found that at 4 years of follow-up (mean = 46.28 months) patients who grazed had less %EWL and more weight regain, and more difficulty in adjusting lifestyle habits, such as following the recommended amount of physical exercise and alcohol intake. Based on 1–12 years of follow-up (mean = 5.8 years), Robinson et al. (2014) found that post-surgical success rate (defined as ≥50% EWL) was higher in those who grazed less frequently vs. those who endorsed grazing more than once a day. Pizato et al. (2017) published a systematic review on the effect of grazing behavior on weight regain after bariatric surgery. The review included 994 patients and a follow-up period ranged from 6 months to 10 years. The prevalence of grazing behavior ranged from 16.6 to 46.6%, and the highest prevalence of significant weight regain was 47%. The authors concluded that their findings supported an association between grazing behavior and weight regain after bariatric surgery, regardless of surgery type and contextual concept of grazing.

6.6.2 Night Eating Syndrome

Night eating syndrome (NES) is conceptualized as a delay in the circadian intake of food, manifested by evening hyperphagia, nocturnal awakenings with ingestion of food, and morning anorexia. Recently, the NES has been included in the DSM-5 as an example of an "other-specified feeding or eating disorder." DSM diagnostic description focuses on *recurrent episodes of night eating, as manifested by eating after awakening from sleep (called nocturnal eating or nocturnal ingestions), or by excessive food consumption after the evening meal (called evening hyperphagia). There is awareness and recall of the eating. The night eating is not better explained by external influences such as changes in the individual's sleep-wake cycle or by local social norms. The night eating causes significant distress and/or impairment in functioning. The disordered pattern of eating is not better explained by binge eating disorder or another mental disorder, including substance use, and is not attributable to another medical disorder or to an effect of medication."* (p. 354).

The most widely used self-assessment measure for screening and for assessing symptom severity is the *Night Eating Questionnaire* (NEQ) developed by Allison et al. (2008). The current version consists of 14 items assessed on a 5-point Likert scale concerning the pattern and timing of food intake, hunger, and cravings for food after the evening meal and during awakenings, mood, and sleep. A score of 25 or greater indicates that the patient needs to be assessed further. At a score of 30 or greater, the positive-predictive value of the NEQ is 72.7%. These parameters were established using a bariatric sample and are therefore relevant to this population.

The prevalence of NES among bariatric candidates varies widely depending on the diagnostic method (range: 8–55%). Several studies have shown a relationship between NES and other abnormal eating patterns including binge eating disorder and loss-of-control eating. In their comprehensive review on the NES in bariatric surgery patients, de Zwaan et al. (2015) concluded that there is no evidence that pre-surgery NES impacts negatively on weight loss after surgery. In a small study of 60 bariatric patients, Ferreira Pinto et al. (2017) reported that improvement of night eating was observed predominantly in patients with pre-operative depressive symptoms and interpreted this finding as consistent with the hypothesis of an important role of mood problems in NES. In a follow-up study of 844 bariatric patients, Nasirzadeh et al. (2018) found that night eating symptoms decreased after surgery and remained lower than baseline throughout follow-up. Yet, the NES score increased significantly between the first and third post-operative years.

6.6.3 Emotional Eating

Emotional eating refers to consuming food in response to emotions such as depression, anxiety, or anger (Nightingale and Cassin 2019). Emotional eating is fairly common among individuals with excess weight, with 37.1% of bariatric surgery candidates endorsing this behavior. Empirical research indicates that individuals with excess weight score higher on measures of emotional eating than those who fall within the normal weight category. The most widely used measure of emotional eating is the *Emotional Eating Scale* (EES), a 25-itemself-report questionnaire designed to assess the tendency of individuals to eat in response to emotions. Higher scores indicate a greater reported desire to eat in response to negative mood states. The EES generates three subscales based upon the mean of items reflecting the urge to eat in response to anger/frustration, anxiety, and depression.

Emotional eating can occur in two different forms: conscious and reflexive (Chesler 2012). Conscious emotional eating reflects the deliberate decision to ease emotional distress through food ingestion. Reflexive emotional eating is an automatic reaction to unrecognized negative feelings. Reflexive emotional eating is reported to be highly associated with alexithymia, a set of cognitive-affective deficits that include difficulties in identifying and communicating feelings, and poor interoceptive awareness, characterized, in part, by difficulty in recognizing and accurately identifying emotions (see Chap. 3). Some evidence suggests that some bariatric candidates might engage in reflexive emotional eating. A study found that morbidly obese females who apply for bariatric surgery reported higher scores on difficulty identifying feelings (alexithymia) and suppression of emotions (interoceptive awareness) than the general population or control group (Zijlstra et al. 2012). Moreover, more negative affect and a higher difficulty identifying feelings were correlated with more emotional eating.

There are limited post-operative data on emotional eating in the literature. In a follow-up study of 844 bariatric patients, Nasirzadeh et al. (2018) found emotional eating subscale scores including EES-anger, EES-anxiety, and EES-depression to significantly decrease after surgery, but increase in the subsequent years. EES scores were not a predictor of post-operative weight loss. These findings align with another study that used the EES to quantify emotional eating and found no statistically significant difference in weight outcome as a result of emotional eating scores 8 months after surgery (Fischer et al. 2007).

6.6.4 Loss-of-Control Eating

Loss-of-control eating refers to eating episodes in which an individual experiences a subjective loss of control during the eating episode, regardless of the amount of food consumed (i.e., it can occur in the absence of overeating). Loss-of-control eating is viewed as an inherent part of binge episodes. For example, adults with obesity and BED experience greater loss of control than those without BED, even after controlling for differences such as negative mood and calories consumed (Nightingale and Cassin 2019). There are no validated scales for measuring loss-of-control eating. However, within the *Eating Disorder Examination Questionnaire* (EDE-Q), there is a subscale assessing the number of times over the last 28 days that the participant reported having lost control while subjectively overeating.

Loss-of-control eating is common among individuals with excess weight, ranging from 22.5% in a sample of women seeking weight loss treatment to 54% among bariatric surgery candidates (Royal et al. 2015). There is preliminary evidence that the persistence of loss-of-control eating after surgery may have detrimental effects on weight outcomes (Fischer et al. 2007; Meany et al. 2014).

6.6.5 Food Addiction

The diagnostic construct of "food addiction" is a highly controversial subject (Fletcher and Kenny 2018). A variety of approaches have been used to measure it, but the *Yale Food Addiction Scale* (YFAS) is currently the best available measure for evaluating food addiction based upon modified DSM criteria for substance use disorders. A food addiction model proposes that some individuals are addicted to certain foods and feel driven to engage in weight-promoting eating behaviors, such as binge eating or compulsive overeating, when exposed to "addictive" food substances. Foods with added fat and refined carbohydrates have been shown to be consumed in a more addictive manner and craved more intensely than less refined foods. Many similarities have been noted between substance use disorders (e.g., alcohol, nicotine) and food addiction, including consuming more of the substance than intended or over a longer period of time, preoccupation with the substance, craving or strong urge to use the substance, and continued consumption despite knowledge of adverse effects (Cassin et al. 2019).

Though some individuals with obesity may display neurological and behavioral similarities to individuals addicted to drugs (Carter et al. 2016), estimates suggest that only approximately 24.9% of overweight/obese individuals report clinically significant symptoms of food addiction and 11.1% of healthy-weight individuals also report these symptoms. Similarly, while food addiction symptoms are associated with binge eating behavior and account for 6–14.8% of the unique variance in binge eating disorder, current estimates suggest that only approximately 56.8% of individuals with binge eating disorder report clinically significant food addiction symptoms. Although there is substantial overlap between food addiction and binge eating symptoms, the two constructs are not synonymous (Gordon et al. 2018).

Ivezaj et al. (2017) published a systematic review of the relationship between food addiction and bariatric surgery. The review was based on 19 studies which assessed food addiction among pre- and/or post-bariatric surgery patients using the YAFS. The presence of food addiction assessed by the YFAS was common among individuals seeking bariatric surgery and was associated with disordered-eating behavior and broad psychopathology. The two studies that prospectively measured food addiction pre- and post-operatively found high levels of food addiction before surgery, which significantly decreased post-surgery. The presence of pre-surgical food addiction was not associated with pre-surgical weight or post-surgical weight outcomes up to 12 months post-surgery; yet, the presence of pre-surgical food addiction was linked to greater pre-operative eating-disorder psychopathology, problematic eating behaviors, and broad levels of psychopathology. The relationship between food addiction and substance misuse was not consistent across different studies.

6.7 Clinical Management

The prevalence of eating disorders among patients seeking bariatric surgery is very high. Pre-surgery assessment should investigate past and/or current symptoms of both major eating disorders (i.e., anorexia nervosa, bulimia nervosa, and binge eating disorder) and other maladaptive eating patterns (i.e., grazing, night eating syndrome, emotional eating, loss-of-control eating, and food addiction). Self-report questionnaire are useful screening tools, especially when combined in a battery that explores the multiple dimensions of eating pathology (loss of control, tendency to restrain, emotional eating, etc.). However, the validity of diagnostic assessment is sometimes weakened by patients' reticence in sharing information that could make them not eligible for bariatric surgery.

Until recently, a pre-operative diagnosis of eating disorder was considered a major contraindication to bariatric surgery. This limitation has been reduced over time and bariatric surgery interventions can now be suitable for selected patients with current eating disorders, even if clinical outcomes and the extent of weight loss depend on the persistence or re-emergence of eating pathology after the intervention. The crucial aspect to consider is that eating pathology is treatable. Recommending pre-operative therapy (medications and/or psychotherapy) and delaying surgery may substantially improve long-term bariatric outcomes. On the other hand, the decision to postpone surgery should be weighed against the risk of loss to follow-up. There is evidence that a significant proportion of patients renounce surgery after a delay recommended on psychological grounds (Sogg et al. 2016).

Post-surgery assessment is as much important as pre-operative diagnostic evaluation, and it should be extended for years after surgery. In most cases, eating pathology and maladaptive eating behaviors decrease significantly during the first year after bariatric surgery. Yet, early remission of disordered eating does not guarantee the complete resolution of these behaviors. Sometimes, eating pathology reemerges in the long run, often in different forms. For example, objective binge eating can turn into subjective binge eating. Because of post-surgery changes in the digestive tract, patients cannot ingest a large amount of food as in objective binge eating but they continue to experience a sense of loss of control over eating much a smaller amount of food, drinking high ealoric fluids, or eating sweets.

KEY POINTS

Eating pathology improves during the first year after surgery. Later on, disordered eating may reemerge, sometimes in different forms.

Post-surgery bulimia and anorexia nervosa are ominous conditions that require quick diagnosis and intervention.

Delaying surgery and treating pre-operative eating pathology improve long-term outcomes.

References

Alger-Mayer S, Rosati C, Polimeni JM, Malone M. Preoperative binge eating status and gastric bypass surgery: a long-term outcome study. Obes Surg. 2009;19(2):139–45. Epub 2008 May 14. PubMed PMID: 18478306. https://doi.org/10.1007/s11695-008-9540-9.

Allison KC, Lundgren JD, O'Reardon JP, Martino NS, Sarwer DB, Wadden TA, Crosby RD, Engel SG, Stunkard AJ. The Night Eating Questionnaire (NEQ): psychometric properties of a measure of severity of the Night Eating Syndrome. Eat Behav. 2008;9(1):62–72. Epub 2007 Mar 28. PubMed PMID: 18167324. https://doi.org/10.1016/j.eatbeh.2007.03.007.

Amianto F, Ottone L, Abbate Daga G, Fassino S. Binge-eating disorder diagnosis and treatment: a recap in front of DSM-5. BMC Psychiatry. 2015;15:70. Review. PubMed PMID: 25885566; PubMed Central PMCID: PMC4397811. https://doi.org/10.1186/s12888-015-0445-6.

Barclay KS, Rushton PW, Forwell SJ. Measurement properties of eating behavior self-assessment tools in adult bariatric surgery populations: a systematic review. Obes Surg. 2015;25(4):720–37. Review. PubMed PMID: 25691348. https://doi.org/10.1007/s11695-015-1593-y.

Brownley KA, Berkman ND, Peat CM, Lohr KN, Cullen KE, Bann CM, Bulik CM. Binge-eating disorder in adults: a systematic review and meta-analysis. Ann Intern Med. 2016;165(6):409–20. Epub 2016 Jun 28. Review. PubMed PMID: 27367316; PubMed Central PMCID: PMC5637727. https://doi.org/10.7326/M15-2455.

Burgmer R, Grigutsch K, Zipfel S, Wolf AM, de Zwaan M, Husemann B, Albus C, Senf W, Herpertz S. The influence of eating behavior and eating pathology on weight loss after gastric restriction operations. Obes Surg. 2005;15(5):684–91. PubMed PMID: 15946461.

Busetto L, Segato G, De Marchi F, Foletto M, De Luca M, Caniato D, Enzi G. Outcome predictors in morbidly obese recipients of an adjustable gastric band. Obes Surg. 2002;12(1):83–92.

Busetto L, Segato G, De Luca M, De Marchi F, Foletto M, Vianello M, Valeri M, Favretti F, Enzi G. Weight loss and postoperative complications in morbidly obese patients with binge eating disorder treated by laparoscopic adjustable gastric banding. Obes Surg. 2005;15(2):195–201. PubMed PMID: 15802061.

Carter A, Hendrikse J, Lee N, Yücel M, Verdejo-Garcia A, Andrews ZB, Hall W. The neurobiology of "Food Addiction" and its implications for obesity treatment and policy. Annu Rev Nutr. 2016;36:105–28. Epub 2016 Jun 1. Review. PubMed PMID: 27296500. https://doi.org/10.1146/annurev-nutr-071715-050909.

Cassin SE, Buchman DZ, Leung SE, Kantarovich K, Hawa A, Carter A, Sockalingam S. Ethical, stigma, and policy implications of food addiction: a scoping review. Nutrients. 2019;11(4):E710. Review. PubMed PMID: 30934743; PubMed Central PMCID: PMC6521112. https://doi.org/10.3390/nu11040710.

Chesler BE. Emotional eating: a virtually untreated risk factor for outcome following bariatric surgery. Scientific World Journal. 2012;2012:365961. Epub 2012 Apr 1. Review. PubMed PMID: 22566765; PubMed Central PMCID: PMC3330752. https://doi.org/10.1100/2012/365961.

Colles SL, Dixon JB, O'Brien PE. Grazing and loss of control related to eating: two high-risk factors following bariatric surgery. Obesity (Silver Spring). 2008;16(3):615–22. Epub 2008 Jan 17. Erratum in: Obesity (Silver Spring). 2011 Nov;19(11):2287. PubMed PMID: 18239603. https://doi.org/10.1038/oby.2007.101.

Conceição EM, Crosby R, Mitchell JE, Engel SG, Wonderlich SA, Simonich HK, Peterson CB, Crow SJ, Le Grange D. Picking or nibbling: frequency and associated clinical features in bulimia nervosa, anorexia nervosa, and binge eating disorder. Int J Eat Disord. 2013;46(8):815–8. Epub 2013 Aug 7. PubMed PMID: 23922133; PubMed Central PMCID: PMC4009470. https://doi.org/10.1002/eat.22167.

Conceição EM, Mitchell JE, Engel SG, Machado PP, Lancaster K, Wonderlich SA. What is "grazing"? Reviewing its definition, frequency, clinical characteristics, and impact on bariatric surgery outcomes, and proposing a standardized definition. Surg Obes Relat Dis. 2014;10(5):973–82. Epub 2014 May 15. Review. PubMed PMID: 25312671. https://doi.org/10.1016/j.soard.2014.05.002.

De Cesare A, Cangemi B, Fiori E, Bononi M, Cangemi R, Basso L. Early and long-term clinical outcomes of bilio-intestinal diversion in morbidly obese patients. Surg Today. 2014;44(8):1424–33.

de Zwaan M, Hilbert A, Swan-Kremeier L, Simonich H, Lancaster K, Howell LM, Mitchell JE. Comprehensive interview assessment of eating behavior 18–35 months after gastric bypass surgery for morbid obesity. Surg Obes Relat Dis. 2010;6(1):79–85.

de Zwaan M, Marschollek M, Allison KC. The Night Eating Syndrome (NES) in bariatric surgery patients. Eur Eat Disord Rev. 2015;23(6):426–34. Epub 2015 Sep 22. Review. PubMed PMID: 26395455. https://doi.org/10.1002/erv.2405.

Deitel M. Anorexia nervosa following bariatric surgery. Obes Surg. 2002;12(6):729–30. PubMed PMID: 12568176.

Ferreira Pinto T, Carvalhedo de Bruin PF, Sales de Bruin VM, Ney Lemos F, Azevedo Lopes FH, Marcos Lopes P. Effects of bariatric surgery on night eating and depressive symptoms: a prospective study. Surg Obes Relat Dis. 2017;13(6):1057–62. Epub 2016 Dec 21. PubMed PMID: 28233690. https://doi.org/10.1016/j.soard.2016.12.010.

Fischer S, Chen E, Katterman S, et al. Emotional eating in a morbidly obese bariatric surgery-seeking population. Obes Surg. 2007;17(6):778–84.

Fletcher PC, Kenny PJ. Food addiction: a valid concept? Neuropsychopharmacology. 2018;43(13):2506–13. Epub 2018 Sep 6. Review. Erratum in: Neuropsychopharmacology. 2018 Dec 7. PubMed PMID: 30188514; PubMed Central PMCID: PMC6224546. https://doi.org/10.1038/s41386-018-0203-9.

Gordon EL, Ariel-Donges AH, Bauman V, Merlo LJ. What is the evidence for "Food Addiction?" A systematic review. Nutrients. 2018;10(4):E477. Review. PubMed PMID: 29649120; PubMed Central PMCID: PMC5946262. https://doi.org/10.3390/nu10040477.

Heriseanu AI, Hay P, Corbit L, Touyz S. Grazing in adults with obesity and eating disorders: a systematic review of associated clinical features and meta-analysis of prevalence. Clin Psychol

Rev. 2017;58:16–32. Epub 2017 Sep 15. Review. PubMed PMID: 28988855. https://doi.org/10.1016/j.cpr.2017.09.004.

Ivezaj V, Wiedemann AA, Grilo CM. Food addiction and bariatric surgery: a systematic review of the literature. Obes Rev. 2017;18(12):1386–97. Epub 2017 Sep 25. Review. PubMed PMID: 28948684; PubMed Central PMCID: PMC5691599. https://doi.org/10.1111/obr.12600.

Ivezaj V, Barnes RD, Cooper Z, Grilo CM. Loss-of-control eating after bariatric/sleeve gastrectomy surgery: Similar to binge-eating disorder despite differences in quantities. Gen Hosp Psychiatry. 2018;54:25–30. Epub 2018 Jul 17. PubMed PMID: 30056316; PubMed Central PMCID: PMC6245943. https://doi.org/10.1016/j.genhosppsych.2018.07.002.

Jones-Corneille LR, Wadden TA, Sarwer DB, Faulconbridge LF, Fabricatore AN, Stack RM, Cottrell FA, Pulcini ME, Webb VL, Williams NN. Axis I psychopathology in bariatric surgery candidates with and without binge eating disorder: results of structured clinical interviews. Obes Surg. 2012;22(3):389–97. PubMed PMID: 21088923; PubMed Central PMCID: PMC3085042. https://doi.org/10.1007/s11695-010-0322-9.

Kofman MD, Lent MR, Swencionis C. Maladaptive eating patterns, quality of life, and weight outcomes following gastric bypass: results of an Internet survey. Obesity (Silver Spring). 2010;18(10):1938–43. Epub 2010 Feb 18. PubMed PMID: 20168309. https://doi.org/10.1038/oby.2010.27.

Mack I, Ölschläger S, Sauer H, von Feilitzsch M, Weimer K, Junne F, Teufel M. Does laparoscopic sleeve gastrectomy improve depression, stress and eating behaviour? A 4-year follow-up study. Obes Surg. 2016;26:2967–73.

Marek RJ, Heinberg LJ, Lavery M, Merrell Rish J, Ashton K. A review of psychological assessment instruments for use in bariatric surgery evaluations. Psychol Assess. 2016;28(9):1142–57. Review. PubMed PMID: 27537008. https://doi.org/10.1037/pas0000286.

Meany G, Conceição E, Mitchell JE. Binge eating, binge eating disorder and loss of control eating: effects on weight outcomes after bariatric surgery. Eur Eat Disord Rev. 2014;22(2):87–91. Review. PubMed PMID: 24347539; PubMed Central PMCID: PMC4420157.

Morseth MS, Hanvold SE, Rø Ø, Risstad H, Mala T, Benth JŠ, Engström M, Olbers T, Henjum S. Self-reported eating disorder symptoms before and after gastric bypass and duodenal switch for super obesity—a 5-year follow-up study. Obes Surg. 2016;26(3):588–94. PubMed PMID: 26173850. https://doi.org/10.1007/s11695-015-1790-8.

Nasirzadeh Y, Kantarovich K, Wnuk S, Okrainec A, Cassin SE, Hawa R, Sockalingam S. Binge eating, loss of control over eating, emotional eating, and night eating after bariatric surgery: results from the Toronto Bari-PSYCH Cohort Study. Obes Surg. 2018;28(7):2032–9. PubMed PMID: 29411241. https://doi.org/10.1007/s11695-018-3137-8.

Nicolau J, Ayala L, Rivera R, Speranskaya A, Sanchís P, Julian X, Fortuny R, Masmiquel L. Postoperative grazing as a risk factor for negative outcomes after bariatric surgery. Eat Behav. 2015;18:147–50. Epub 2015 Jun 6. PubMed PMID: 26094133. https://doi.org/10.1016/j.eatbeh.2015.05.008.

Niego SH, Kofman MD, Weiss JJ, Geliebter A. Binge eating in the bariatric surgery population: a review of the literature. Int J Eat Disord. 2007;40(4):349–59. Review. PubMed PMID: 17304586.

Nightingale BA, Cassin SE. Disordered eating among individuals with excess weight: a review of recent research. Curr Obes Rep. 2019;8(2):112–27. Review. PubMed PMID: 30827011. https://doi.org/10.1007/s13679-019-00333-5.

Parker K, Brennan L. Measurement of disordered eating in bariatric surgery candidates: a systematic review of the literature. Obes Res Clin Pract. 2015;9(1):12–25. Epub 2014 Feb 28. Review. PubMed PMID: 25660171. https://doi.org/10.1016/j.orcp.2014.01.005.

Parker K, Mitchell S, O'Brien P, Brennan L. Psychometric evaluation of disordered eating measures in bariatric surgery candidates. Obes Surg. 2016;26(3):563–75. PubMed PMID: 26163361. https://doi.org/10.1007/s11695-015-1780-x.

Pizato N, Botelho PB, Gonçalves VSS, Dutra ES, de Carvalho KMB. Effect of grazing behavior on weight regain post-bariatric surgery: a systematic review. Nutrients. 2017;9(12):E1322. .

Review. PubMed PMID: 29206132; PubMed Central PMCID: PMC5748772. https://doi.org/10.3390/nu9121322.

Poole NA, Al Atar A, Kuhanendran D, Bidlake L, Fiennes A, McCluskey S, Morgan JF. Compliance with surgical after-care following bariatric surgery for morbid obesity: a retrospective study. Obes Surg. 2005;15(2):261–5. https://doi.org/10.1381/0960892053268499.

Pucci A, Cheung WH, Jones J, Manning S, Kingett H, Adamo M, Elkalaawy M, Jenkinson A, Finer N, Doyle J, Hashemi M, Batterham RL. A case of severe anorexia, excessive weight loss and high peptide YY levels after sleeve gastrectomy. Endocrinol Diabetes Metab Case Rep. 2015;2015:150020. Epub 2015 Jun 1. PubMed PMID: 26664728; PubMed Central PMCID: PMC4674657. https://doi.org/10.1530/EDM-15-0020.

Robinson AH, Adler S, Stevens HB, Darcy AM, Morton JM, Safer DL. What variables are associated with successful weight loss outcomes for bariatric surgery after 1 year? Surg Obes Relat Dis. 2014;10(4):697–704.

Royal S, Wnuk S, Warwick K, Hawa R, Sockalingam S. Night eating and loss of control over eating in bariatric surgery candidates. J Clin Psychol Med Settings. 2015;22(1):14–9. PubMed PMID: 25450651. https://doi.org/10.1007/s10880-014-9411-6.

Saunders R. Post-surgery group therapy for gastric bypass patients. Obes Surg. 2004;14(8):1128–31. Review. PubMed PMID: 15479605.

Segal A, Kinoshita Kussunoki D, Larino MA. Post-surgical refusal to eat: anorexia nervosa, bulimia nervosa or a new eating disorder? A case series. Obes Surg. 2004;14(3):353–60. PubMed PMID: 15072657.

Sekuła M, Boniecka I, Paśnik K. Bulimia nervosa in obese patients qualified for bariatric surgery—clinical picture, background and treatment. Wideochir Inne Tech Maloinwazyjne. 2019;14(3):408–14. Epub 2019 Jan 16. Review. PubMed PMID: 31534571; PubMed Central PMCID: PMC6748054. https://doi.org/10.5114/wiitm.2019.81312.

Shear M, DeFilippis EM. Complications of pre-operative anorexia nervosa in bariatric surgery. Obes Res Clin Pract. 2015;9(4):424–8. Epub 2015 Feb 27. PubMed PMID: 25736337. https://doi.org/10.1016/j.orcp.2015.02.008.

Sogg S, Lauretti J, West-Smith L. Recommendations for the presurgical psychosocial evaluation of bariatric surgery patients. Surg Obes Relat Dis. 2016;12(4):731–49. Epub 2016 Feb 12. Review. PubMed PMID: 27179400. https://doi.org/10.1016/j.soard.2016.02.008.

Tess BH, Maximiano-Ferreira L, Pajecki D, Wang YP. Bariatric surgery and binge eating disorder: should surgeons care about it? A literature review of prevalence and assessment tools. Arq Gastroenterol. 2019;56(1):55–60. Review. PubMed PMID: 31141066. https://doi.org/10.1590/S0004-2803.201900000-10.

Tortorella A, Volpe U, Fabrazzo M, Tolone S, Docimo L, Monteleone P. From over- to underweight: treatment of post-surgical anorexia nervosa in morbid obesity. Eat Weight Disord. 2015;20(4):529–32. Epub 2015 Apr 22. PubMed PMID: 25900088. https://doi.org/10.1007/s40519-015-0192-1.

Ward K, Citrome L. Lisdexamfetamine: chemistry, pharmacodynamics, pharmacokinetics, and clinical efficacy, safety, and tolerability in the treatment of binge eating disorder. Expert Opin Drug Metab Toxicol. 2018;14(2):229–38. Epub 2018 Jan 4. Review. PubMed PMID: 29258368. https://doi.org/10.1080/17425255.2018.1420163.

Yashkov YI, Bekuzarov DK. Effectiveness of biliopancreatic diversion in the patients with bulimia nervosa. Obes Surg. 2006;16(11):1433–9. PubMed PMID: 17132407.

Zijlstra H, van Middendorp H, Devaere L, Larsen JK, van Ramshorst B, Geenen R. Emotion processing and regulation in women with morbid obesity who apply for bariatric surgery. Psychol Health. 2012;27(12):1375–87. Epub 2011 Jul 22. PubMed PMID: 21777156. https://doi.org/10.1080/08870446.2011.600761.

Depressive Disorders

7

Abstract

Depression is one of the most common pre-operative psychiatric conditions among bariatric surgery candidates. In some studies, pre-surgical assessment showed that the percentage of patients suffering from depression is around 40%. There is evidence for short- and medium-term improvement in depressive symptoms after surgery. However, a subgroup of patients exhibits erosion of these improvements or new onset of depression in the long run. Findings on the impact of pre-operative depression on the outcome of bariatric surgery are mixed. The assessment of long-term outcomes should not be limited to weight loss. Future studies should clarify if pre-operative depression predicts other negative outcomes, including increased suicide risk, and greater vulnerability to substance abuse and/or maladaptive eating patterns. Even if mild and moderate depression is not a contraindication for bariatric surgery, therapy should be offered to bariatric candidates who present depressive symptoms during the pre-operative assessment. For some patients, pre-surgery mental health screening may be the first and only opportunity to become aware of their mood disturbance and to be informed about therapeutic options.

Keywords

Depression · Screening · Differential diagnosis · Pre-surgery prevalence Post-surgery course · Relapse · New onset

© Springer Nature Switzerland AG 2020
A. Troisi, *Bariatric Psychology and Psychiatry*,
https://doi.org/10.1007/978-3-030-44834-9_7

7.1   Background

Clinically significant depressive symptoms are prevalent in individuals with obesity and significantly contribute to illness burden. A reciprocal link has been demonstrated to exist between obesity and depression, wherein obese individuals are at a higher risk for depression and depressed patients are at higher risk for obesity (Luppino et al. 2010; Ambrósio et al. 2018). Thus, it is understandable why depression is one of the most common pre-operative psychiatric conditions among bariatric surgery candidates. The overall rate of depression varies with diagnostic methods (standardized interviews versus rating scales), but, in some studies, pre-surgical assessment showed that the percentage of bariatric surgery candidates suffering from depression is around 40%. Diagnosing depression and assessing the severity of depressive symptoms is clinically relevant both before and after bariatric surgery. In some cases, pre-operative depression is a predictor of negative outcomes. In other cases, depression improves after surgery and does not negatively impact post-operative outcomes.

7.2   Basic Notions

In psychiatry and clinical psychology, the term "depression" is used to indicate both a syndrome and an individual symptom. It is important to consider such a difference when reporting the results of mental health assessment of bariatric patients. Depression as a syndrome includes a group of depressive disorders characterized by persistent low mood, loss of pleasure, lack of energy, and a variable combination of emotional, cognitive, and somatic symptoms. DSM-5 diagnostic criteria for major depressive disorder (its term for clinical depression) require the presence of one core symptom, either low mood or anhedonia (i.e., loss of pleasure or enjoyment in formerly pleasurable activities). Associated emotional symptoms may include reduced self-esteem and self-confidence, ideas of guilt and worthlessness, and feelings of hopelessness regarding the future. Associated cognitive symptoms may include reduced concentration and attention, and diminished ability to think. Associated somatic symptoms may include psychomotor agitation and/or retardation, reduced sleep, appetite, and libido. There is often a sleep pattern of early waking and maximal lowering of mood in the morning. In the most severe cases, psychotic symptoms (i.e., delusions and/or hallucinations) may be present.

The lifetime risk of depression is between 10 and 20% (US national data), with rates almost doubled in women (Hasin et al. 2018). Onset is most common in the third decade. Depressive disorders are among the leading causes of disability worldwide. Depression as a symptom is a common manifestation of a variety of psychiatric and medical conditions. Even when the symptoms described are very typical of depression, it is always important to consider other differential diagnoses. The mental health assessment of bariatric patients presenting with depression should always explore the possibility of alternative diagnoses (Table 7.1). Probably, the most critical differential diagnosis is between depression and bipolar disorder.

Table 7.1 Differential diagnosis of depression in bariatric candidates

DIAGNOSIS	CLINICAL FEATURES	BARIATRIC IMPLICATIONS
Psychotic depression	Hallucinations and/or delusions	Bariatric surgery contraindicated
Bipolar depression	History of hypomania or mania	Management as in bipolar disorder
Dysthymia	Chronic, moderate severity	Indication for pre-and post-operative psychotherapy
Atypical depression	Reversed somatic symptoms	Associated with overeating
Eating disorder	Depression secondary to eating symptoms	Focus on eating symptoms
Personality disorder	Dysfunctional personality traits	Focus on personality traits
Substance abuse	Depression secondary to substance use	Bariatric surgery contraindicated

7.3   Bariatric Data

7.3.1   Prevalence

Compared to the general population, bariatric patients have a higher prevalence of depressive disorders. Dawes et al. (2016) published a meta-analysis including 59 studies and 65,363 patients to determine the pre-operative point prevalence of mental health conditions among bariatric surgery candidates and recipients. Depression was the most common individual diagnosis. The prevalence of depression (19%) was greater than in the general US population (8%). Although the size of the meta-analysis in terms of both the number of studies included and patients enrolled makes the Dawes et al.'s study a landmark reference, the combination of diagnostic data based on rating scales or structured interviews complicates the interpretation of the findings. Studies based on structured interviews (the best diagnostic method) have yielded different prevalence rates. A study conducted in Germany with face-to-face (SCID-I) interviews of 107 bariatric surgery candidates found that the majority of participants presented with lifetime depressive disorders (56.1%) and one third met criteria for current depressive disorders (32.7%) (de Zwaan et al. 2011). Interviewing 393 Brazilian bariatric surgery candidates with the SCID-I, Duarte-Guerra et al. (2015) reported a lifetime prevalence of major depression of 27.5% (current prevalence: 7.9%). Malik et al. (2014) reported the lifetime and current prevalence rates of psychiatric disorders in 1089 bariatric surgery candidates diagnosed with structured interviews in 5 different studies. Current prevalence rates for depression (major depression or dysthymia) ranged from 6.4 to 31.5%. Lifetime prevalence rates ranged from 22 to 54.8%. Overall, these findings show that many patients seeking bariatric surgery have a depressive disorder and many more have suffered from depression in the past, which implies an increased risk of post-operative relapse.

7.3.2 Post-operative Course

The impact of bariatric surgery on depression is under debate. The prospective study by de Zwaan et al. (2011) based on structured interviews found a progressive decrease of the point prevalence of depressive disorders after bariatric surgery: baseline, 32.7%; 6–12 months post-surgery, 16.5%; 24–36% months post-surgery, 14.3%. The authors emphasized that, although bariatric surgery was associated with the improvement of depressive symptoms, a substantial number of patients remained depressed as indicated by a post-surgery prevalence rate much higher than that of the general population. A recent systematic review assessed the short- (<24 months) and long-term (>24 months) effects of bariatric surgery on depression (Gill et al. 2019). Fourteen prospective studies were included in the review. There was a large disparity in sample size (range: 21 to 1097 participants). Studies included in the review found statistically significant reductions in depressive symptoms following the first 24 months after surgery. The largest reductions were seen in depressive symptoms within the first 2 years following surgery. Depressive symptoms did begin to rise after the first 2 years, but most studies maintained statistically significant reductions compared to baseline. Using the National Health Insurance Research Database of Taiwan, Lu et al. (2018) identified 2302 patients who underwent bariatric surgery in 2001–2009. These patients were matched by propensity score to 6493 obese patients who did not receive bariatric surgery. The surgical and control cohorts were followed until death, for any diagnosis of major depressive disorder or 31 December 2012, whichever came first. The study found a significant 1.50-fold increase in the risk of major depression in the surgical group compared with the control group. In addition, the risk of major depression increased 2.36-fold with the malabsorptive type of surgery and 1.38-fold with the restrictive type of surgery compared with controls, implying that malabsorption plays a more important role than restricted food intake in major depression development. It was also found that the incidence of major depression increased 4 years after surgery compared with the incidence in controls.

Several hypotheses have been advanced to explain the post-operative course of depression after bariatric surgery. Initial improvement may be related to physiological (e.g., decreased levels of pro-inflammatory cytokines involved in the pathogenesis of depression) and/or psychological (e.g., enhanced self-esteem) mechanisms triggered by massive weight loss. Later reemergence of depression may be related to weight regain or the occurrence of medical comorbidities. Another possible factor is altered pharmacotherapy. The absorption of antidepressant medications may decrease substantially, causing exacerbation of symptoms in post-bariatric patients who are on drug treatment for depression. Compared to pre-surgery levels, maximum serum levels of escitalopram, sertraline, and duloxetine have been reported to decrease after Roux-en-Y gastric bypass. With no adjustment of medication dose, the risk of suicide may increase due to inadequate treatment.

Müller et al. (2019) have reasonably summarized the status of current knowledge on the impact of bariatric surgery on depression as follows: *Considerable evidence shows short- and medium-term improvement in depressive symptoms after surgery. However, a subgroup of patients exhibits erosion of these improvements or new onset of depression in the long run.* (p. 84).

7.3.3 Impact on Outcome

Few studies have investigated the impact of pre-operative depression on the outcome of bariatric surgery. Some studies based on small samples reported a negative association between baseline depression and post-operative weigh loss. For example, De Zwaan et al. (2011) found that the presence of a depressive disorder was significantly associated with a lower degree of weight loss at 24–36 months, but not at 6–12 months ($n = 107$). However, in their recent review, Gill et al. (2019) concluded that pre-operative depression scores did not predict outcomes of post-operative BMI. These findings are encouraging, but the assessment of long-term outcomes should not be limited to total weight loss, weight loss maintenance, and weight regain. Future studies should clarify if pre-operative depression predicts other negative outcomes, including increased suicide risk, and greater vulnerability to substance abuse, and/or maladaptive eating patterns (e.g., emotional eating or food addiction).

7.4 Assessment

Considering the high prevalence of depression among bariatric surgery candidates, pre-operative assessment should always include an accurate investigation of current and past depressive symptoms. There are many questionnaires that can be used for the screening of depression, including the *Beck Depression Inventory* (BDI), the *Patient Health Questionnaire-9* (PHQ-9), the *Montgomery-Åsberg Depression Rating Scale* (MADRS), and the *Hamilton Depression Rating Scale* (HDRS) (Alabi et al. 2018; Ayloo et al. 2015; Duarte-Guerra et al. 2016; Ivezaj et al. 2016; Kroenke et al. 2001; Schutt et al. 2016; Srivatsan et al. 2018). The MADRS and the HDRS are clinician-rated instruments whereas the BDI and the PHQ-9 are self-report scales.

The 21-item BDI assess all DSM diagnostic symptoms of depression and additional symptoms (e.g., irritability). A large proportion of BDI items focus on the cognitive symptoms of depression, such as self-esteem, guilt, feeling disappointed in oneself, feeling of being punished, and pessimism. As a result, cognitive symptoms of depression contribute disproportionately to the BDI score. Each item is composed of four first-person statements graded by the degree of depression severity it typically represents and rated on a 4-point ordinal scale (0 to 3). The total BDI score is calculated by summing the 21 items and can range from 0 to 63. The PHQ-9 is the depression module of the Patient Health Questionnaire, a self-report version of the PRIME-MD diagnostic instrument for common mental disorders. The score of each of the 9 items ranges from 0 to 3, with item 9 screening for the presence of suicide ideation. The MADRS is a 10-item clinician-rated scale assessing different symptoms of depression. Sad mood is assessed by two items that capture the observer perspective and reported subjective experience, respectively. The other eight items assess tension, sleep, appetite, concentration, lassitude (activity), inability to feel (anhedonia), pessimism, and suicidal thoughts. Each item is rated on a 7-point (0 to 6) ordinal scale. A total score is computed as the sum of the 10 items and can range from 0 to 60. Higher scores reflect more severe depression. The 17-item HDRS assesses mood, guilt, suicidal thoughts, early insomnia, middle insomnia, late insomnia, activity, psychomotor retardation, agitation, psychic anxiety, somatic anxiety, appetite, fatigue, libido, hypochondriasis, weight loss, and insight. Nine items are scored on a 5-point (0 to 4) ordinal scale, and eight items are scored on a 3-point (0, 1, 2) scale. A total score is calculated as the sum of the 17 items and can range from 0 to 52. Higher scores reflect more severe depression. The relatively large number of items assessing sleep, appetite, weight loss, libido, and fatigue mean that somatic symptoms contribute disproportionately to the total score. For this reason, the HDRS may not be suitable for an obese population due to the overlap between somatic symptoms of depression and physical symptoms related to obesity.

Questionnaires are screening tools, not diagnostic instruments. The ideal assessment procedure should be based on the administration of one screening questionnaire followed by structured interviews of those patients who score higher than the cut-off score for that questionnaire. Structured interviews are costly and put additional requirements on clinicians' training and consultation times. However, they offer several advantages over questionnaires including categorical diagnosis of depressive disorders, differential diagnosis with other psychiatric disorders presenting with depressive symptoms, and the identification of comorbid psychiatric disorders. Among bariatric candidates, depressive disorders are highly comorbid with eating disorders; and, in the general population, many cases of bipolar disorder and personality disorders may be misdiagnosed as depressive disorders.

Post-operative assessment of depressive symptoms and depressive disorders is crucial for minimizing negative outcomes (e.g., alcohol abuse and weight regain) and suicide risk. Long-term post-operative assessment is as much important as pre-operative assessment. Although the majority of bariatric patients show short- and medium-term improvement in depressive symptoms after surgery, only long-term follow-up can detect the persistence or re-emergence of depressive disorders. How long should the follow-up last is not clear. Surely, the period of 2 years monitored by most studies is too short. For example, (Booth et al. 2015) reported that, at the 7-year follow-up, the percentage of post-bariatric patients with clinical depression was 37%, a number identical to the pre-operative prevalence (36%). Out of 1097 participants, 1065 were taking antidepressant drugs at the 5-year follow-up, a number surpassing pre-surgery prescription levels.

> **ASSESSMENT TIPS**
>
> Considering the high prevalence of depression among bariatric surgery candidates, pre-operative assessment should always include an accurate investigation of current and past depressive symptoms.
>
> Patients scoring positive on screening questionnaires should be interviewed.
>
> Structured interview should focus on differential diagnosis and psychiatric comorbidity.
>
> Patients with a history of mood disorders need post-operative long-term follow-up.

7.5   Clinical Management

Depression is a treatable condition that can improve with psychological and/or pharmacological interventions. Even if mild and moderate depression is not a contraindication for bariatric surgery, therapy should be offered to bariatric candidates who present depressive symptoms during the pre-operative assessment. For some patients, pre-surgery mental health screening may be the first and only opportunity to become aware of their mood disturbance and to be informed about therapeutic options. If the patient agrees on being treated, bariatric surgery may be postponed until remission of depressive symptoms (which generally takes 2–4 months). Gade et al. (2015) conducted a randomized controlled trial to ascertain whether a pre-operative 10-week cognitive behavioral therapy (CBT) intervention exceeded usual care in the improvement of dysfunctional eating behaviors, mood, affective symptoms, and body weight 1 year after bariatric surgery. There was a significant reduction in depressive symptoms in the CBT group between T0 (baseline) and T1 (post CBT/pre-operatively) and between T1 and T2 (1 year after surgery). However, there was no difference in weight loss at T2 between the CBT group and the control group. A more recent report from the same research group showed that pre-operative group psychotherapy resulted in short-term reduction in depressive symptoms but the effect disappeared 4 years after surgery (Hjelmesæth et al. 2019).

There is a paucity of studies investigating treatment for post-operative bariatric surgery patients suffering from depression. The Bariatric Surgery and Education (BaSE) study aimed to assess the efficacy of a psychoeducational group program following surgery in addition to conventional postoperative visits. Three years post-surgery, patients with clinically relevant depression scores at baseline assigned to the BaSE program reported lower depression scores, better health-related quality of life, and a trend toward more weight loss compared to the control group (Wild et al. 2017). In conclusion, preliminary evidence suggests that pre- and post-operative psychotherapy, and in particular CBT, may lead to significant and meaningful benefits in bariatric patients' psychological well-being.

KEY POINTS

Depression is one of the most common pre-operative psychiatric conditions among bariatric surgery candidates.

Most patients show short- and medium-term improvement in depressive symptoms after surgery. However, in the long run, relapsing or new onset depression may occur.

Preliminary evidence shows that pre-operative depression does not negatively impact surgery outcomes.

Elevated risk for post-surgery development or reoccurrence of depression implies the need for monitoring vulnerable patients.

References

Alabi F, Guilbert L, Villalobos G, Mendoza K, Hinojosa R, Melgarejo JC, Espinosa O, Sepúlveda EM, Zerrweck C. Depression before and after bariatric surgery in low-income patients: the utility of the beck depression inventory. Obes Surg. 2018;28(11):3492–8. PubMed PMID: 29984375. https://doi.org/10.1007/s11695-018-3371-0.

Ambrósio G, Kaufmann FN, Manosso L, Platt N, Ghisleni G, Rodrigues ALS, Rieger DK, Kaster MP. Depression and peripheral inflammatory profile of patients with obesity. Psychoneuroendocrinology. 2018;91:132–41. Epub 2018 Mar 9. Review. PubMed PMID: 29550676. https://doi.org/10.1016/j.psyneuen.2018.03.005.

Ayloo S, Thompson K, Choudhury N, Sheriffdeen R. Correlation between the Beck Depression Inventory and bariatric surgical procedures. Surg Obes Relat Dis. 2015;11(3):637–42. Epub 2014 Nov 13. PubMed PMID: 25863536. https://doi.org/10.1016/j.soard.2014.11.005.

Booth H, Khan O, Prevost AT, Reddy M, Charlton J, Gulliford MC. King's Bariatric Surgery Study Group. Impact of bariatric surgery on clinical depression. Interrupted time series study with matched controls. J Affect Disord. 2015;174:644–9. https://doi.org/10.1016/j.jad.2014.12.050. Epub 2014 Dec 29. PubMed PMID: 25577158.

Dawes AJ, Maggard-Gibbons M, Maher AR, Booth MJ, Miake-Lye I, Beroes JM, Shekelle PG. Mental health conditions among patients seeking and undergoing bariatric surgery: a meta-analysis. JAMA. 2016;315(2):150–63. PubMed PMID: 26757464. https://doi.org/10.1001/jama.2015.18118.

de Zwaan M, Enderle J, Wagner S, Mühlhans B, Ditzen B, Gefeller O, Mitchell JE, Müller A. Anxiety and depression in bariatric surgery patients: a prospective, follow-up study using structured clinical interviews. J Affect Disord. 2011;133(1-2):61–8. Epub 2011 Apr 17. PubMed PMID: 21501874. https://doi.org/10.1016/j.jad.2011.03.025.

Duarte-Guerra LS, Coêlho BM, Santo MA, Wang YP. Psychiatric disorders among obese patients seeking bariatric surgery: results of structured clinical interviews. Obes Surg. 2015;25(5):830–7. PubMed PMID: 25358821. https://doi.org/10.1007/s11695-014-1464-y.

Duarte-Guerra LS, Gorenstein C, Paiva-Medeiros PF, Santo MA, Lotufo Neto F, Wang YP. Clinical utility of the Montgomery-Åsberg Depression Rating Scale for the detection of depression among bariatric surgery candidates. BMC Psychiatry. 2016;16:119. PubMed PMID: 27138750; PubMed Central PMCID: PMC4852448. https://doi.org/10.1186/s12888-016-0823-8.

Gade H, Friborg O, Rosenvinge JH, Småstuen MC, Hjelmesæth J. The impact of a preoperative cognitive behavioural therapy (CBT) on dysfunctional eating behaviours, affective symptoms and body weight 1 year after bariatric surgery: a randomised controlled trial. Obes Surg.

2015;25(11):2112–9. PubMed PMID: 25893651; PubMed Central PMCID: PMC4595536. https://doi.org/10.1007/s11695-015-1673-z.

Gill H, Kang S, Lee Y, Rosenblat JD, Brietzke E, Zuckerman H, McIntyre RS. The long-term effect of bariatric surgery on depression and anxiety. J Affect Disord. 2019;246:886–94. Epub 2018 Dec 28. PubMed PMID: 30795495. https://doi.org/10.1016/j.jad.2018.12.113.

Hasin DS, Sarvet AL, Meyers JL, Saha TD, Ruan WJ, Stohl M, Grant BF. Epidemiology of adult DSM-5 major depressive disorder and its specifiers in the United States. JAMA Psychiat. 2018;75(4):336–46. PubMed PMID: 29450462; PubMed Central PMCID: PMC5875313. https://doi.org/10.1001/jamapsychiatry.2017.4602.

Hjelmesæth J, Rosenvinge JH, Gade H, Friborg O. Effects of cognitive behavioral therapy on eating behaviors, affective symptoms, and weight loss after bariatric surgery: a randomized clinical trial. Obes Surg. 2019;29(1):61–9. PubMed PMID: 30112603; PubMed Central PMCID: PMC6320349. https://doi.org/10.1007/s11695-018-3471-x.

Ivezaj V, Barnes RD, Grilo CM. Validity and clinical utility of subtyping by the Beck Depression Inventory in women seeking gastric bypass surgery. Obes Surg. 2016;26(9):2068–73. PubMed PMID: 26762280; PubMed Central PMCID: PMC5129658. https://doi.org/10.1007/s11695-016-2047-x.

Kroenke K, Spitzer RL, Williams JB. The PHQ-9: validity of a brief depression severity measure. J Gen Intern Med. 2001;16(9):606–13. PubMed PMID: 11556941; PubMed Central PMCID: PMC1495268.

Lu CW, Chang YK, Lee YH, Kuo CS, Chang HH, Huang CT, Hsu CC, Huang KC. Increased risk for major depressive disorder in severely obese patients after bariatric surgery—a 12-year nationwide cohort study. Ann Med. 2018;50(7):605–12. Epub 2018 Sep 7. PubMed PMID: 30101619. https://doi.org/10.1080/07853890.2018.1511917.

Luppino FS, de Wit LM, Bouvy PF, Stijnen T, Cuijpers P, Penninx BW, Zitman FG. Overweight, obesity, and depression: a systematic review and meta-analysis of longitudinal studies. Arch Gen Psychiatry. 2010;67(3):220–9. Review. PubMed PMID: 20194822. https://doi.org/10.1001/archgenpsychiatry.2010.2.

Malik S, Mitchell JE, Engel S, Crosby R, Wonderlich S. Psychopathology in bariatric surgery candidates: a review of studies using structured diagnostic interviews. Compr Psychiatry. 2014;55(2):248–59. Epub 2013 Oct 24. Review. PubMed PMID: 24290079; PubMed Central PMCID: PMC3985130. https://doi.org/10.1016/j.comppsych.2013.08.021.

Müller A, Hase C, Pommnitz M, de Zwaan M. Depression and suicide after bariatric surgery. Curr Psychiatry Rep. 2019;21(9):84. Review. PubMed PMID: 31410656. https://doi.org/10.1007/s11920-019-1069-1.

Schutt PE, Kung S, Clark MM, Koball AM, Grothe KB. Comparing the Beck Depression Inventory-II (BDI-II) and Patient Health Questionnaire (PHQ-9) depression measures in an Outpatient Bariatric Clinic. Obes Surg. 2016;26(6):1274–8. PubMed PMID: 26341087. https://doi.org/10.1007/s11695-015-1877-2.

Srivatsan S, Guduguntla V, Young KZ, Arastu A, Strong CR, Cassidy R, Ghaferi AA. Clinical versus patient-reported measures of depression in bariatric surgery. Surg Endosc. 2018;32(8):3683–90. Epub 2018 Feb 12. PubMed PMID: 29435747. https://doi.org/10.1007/s00464-018-6101-8.

Wild B, Hünnemeyer K, Sauer H, Schellberg D, Müller-Stich BP, Königsrainer A, Weiner R, Zipfel S, Herzog W, Teufel M. Sustained effects of a psychoeducational group intervention following bariatric surgery: follow-up of the randomized controlled BaSE study. Surg Obes Relat Dis. 2017;13(9):1612–8. Epub 2017 Apr 1. PubMed PMID: 28551374. https://doi.org/10.1016/j.soard.2017.03.034.

Anxiety Disorders, OCD, and PTSD

8

Abstract

Studies of pathological anxiety in bariatric patients often combine data on anxiety disorders with data on obsessive-compulsive disorder (OCD) or post-traumatic stress disorder (PTSD). Among bariatric patients, the prevalence rate of anxiety disorders is high. According to the majority of prospective studies, when successful outcome is measured in terms of weight loss, the impact of pre-operative anxiety seems to be negligible. Outcome measures other than weight loss offer a different perspective. Pre-operative anxiety correlates with post-operative anxiety and predicts an increased utilization of mental health services and poorer quality of life after surgery. Unlike depressive symptoms, anxiety symptoms do not improve substantially after bariatric surgery, not even when post-operative assessment is made in the short term. There are few data on the post-surgery course of OCD or the prognostic value of OCD for surgery outcome. PTSD symptoms predict non-completion of the pre-surgery assessment and tend to persist after surgery.

Keywords

Anxiety disorders · Obsessive-compulsive disorder · Post-traumatic stress disorders · Quality of life

8.1 Background

Anxiety disorders are the most common and chronic mental disorders among patients seeking surgical treatment for obesity. Because of their presumed low severity and modest disabling impact on daily life, this class of psychiatric disorders has been relatively overlooked by clinicians who take care of bariatric patients (Duarte-Guerra et al. 2015). Paying scarce attention to anxiety symptoms in

© Springer Nature Switzerland AG 2020
A. Troisi, *Bariatric Psychology and Psychiatry*,
https://doi.org/10.1007/978-3-030-44834-9_8

bariatric patients reflects the fact that, more in general, the association between anxiety and obesity has been investigated less thoroughly compared to the association between depression and obesity.

Studies of pathological anxiety in bariatric patients often combine data on anxiety disorders with data on obsessive-compulsive disorder (OCD) or post-traumatic stress disorder (PTSD), although these two conditions are classified apart in DSM-5. For this reason, and because the data on OCD and PTSD are so few that they do not deserve separate discussion, this chapter outlines basic notions on the diagnostic classification and clinical features of anxiety disorders, OCD, and PTSD; illustrates assessment procedures for measuring symptom severity; and reviews published data on the prevalence, outcomes, and management of anxiety disorders, OCD, and PTSD in bariatric surgery patients.

8.2   Basic Notions

8.2.1   Anxiety Disorders

DSM-5 classification of anxiety disorders include 10 different syndromes, some of which are not relevant to bariatric psychiatry (e.g., selective mutism or separation anxiety disorder) and will not be described here. Major anxiety disorders are generalized anxiety disorder, panic disorder, and phobias (specific phobia, social anxiety disorder, and agoraphobia). In the current version of the DSM, obsessive-compulsive disorder is classified apart from anxiety disorders but most studies of bariatric patients did not make such a distinction.

Generalized anxiety disorder is characterized by generalized, persistent, excessive anxiety, worry, and feelings of apprehension about a number of life situations that the patient finds difficult to control, lasting 6 months or longer. Psychological manifestations of anxiety (e.g., being startled, concentration difficulty, sleep problems) are associated with symptoms of autonomic arousal (e.g., palpitations, tremor, dry mouth). Generalized anxiety disorder may be comorbid with other anxiety disorders, depression, or alcohol and drug abuse. Panic disorder is characterized by episodic and recurrent attacks of severe panic which occur unpredictably and are not restricted to any particular situation. Panic attacks consist of both mental (e.g., fear of dying or going crazy, derealization, depersonalization) and physical (e.g., chest pain, palpitations, dizziness, trembling) symptoms typically lasting only a few minutes. Phobia is an intense and irrational fear of an object, situation, place, or person that is recognized as excessive or unreasonable. Specific phobia consists of marked fear and avoidance of a specific object (e.g., snakes) or situation (e.g., tunnels) other than those feared in social phobia or agoraphobia. Social anxiety disorder (also named social phobia) is characterized by a persistent fear of social situations in which the individual is exposed to unfamiliar people or to possible scrutiny by others and fears that he or she will be humiliated or embarrassed (e.g., by blushing or vomiting). Agoraphobia is characterized by fear and avoidance of places and situations from which escape may be difficult or in which help may not be available in the event of having a panic attack.

There are many psychometric instruments designed for assessing anxiety, some of which focus on symptoms of specific anxiety disorders (e.g., panic disorder or social phobia). Among the instruments measuring anxiety in general, the *Hospital Anxiety and Depression Scale* (HADS) was designed to provide a simple yet reliable tool for use in medical practice. The HADS only takes 2–5 min to complete and includes two independent subscales for measuring anxiety and depression. On each subscale, total score can range from 0 to 21, with a score of 0 to 7 being in the normal range and a score of 11 or higher indicating probable presence of clinical symptoms. The HADS gives less weight to somatic symptoms relative to cognitive and affective symptoms, which is an advantage in bariatric patients.

The three main anxiety disorders (panic disorder, generalized anxiety disorder, and social phobia) are treated with psychotherapy (e.g., individual or group cognitive-behavioral therapy (CBT), relaxation, psychodynamic therapies), medications (selective serotonin reuptake inhibitors (SSRIs), benzodiazepines, tricyclic antidepressants), or a combination of the two. A meta-analysis of 234 randomized-controlled studies involving 37,333 patients found that medications were more effective than psychotherapies (Bandelow et al. 2015).

8.2.2   OCD

OCD is characterized by recurrent obsessions and compulsions. Obsessions are unwanted intrusive thoughts, images, or urges that repeatedly enter the patient's mind (e.g., excessive concern with order or symmetry, fear of jumping in front of a train). Patients attempt to suppress them and recognize them as absurd and a product of their own mind. Compulsions are repetitive, purposeful, physical, or mental behaviors performed with reluctance in response to an obsession (e.g., counting, checking, rearrangement of objects to achieve symmetry). OCD is ranked by the World Health Organization as one of the ten most disabling illnesses in terms of impact on quality of life. The *Yale-Brown Obsessive Compulsive Scale* (Y-BOCS) is the most widely used psychometric instrument to measure symptom severity. Approved treatments include cognitive behavioral therapy combined with exposure and response prevention (CBT-ERP) and drug therapy with SSRIs and/or clomipramine.

8.2.3   PTSD

PTSD is an intense, prolonged, delayed reaction following exposure to an exceptionally traumatic event (e.g., physical assault, sexual abuse, natural disaster). PTSD symptoms must occur within 6 months of the event and include reliving the situation (e.g., persistent intrusive thinking of the trauma and flashbacks), avoiding reminders of trauma, hyperarousal (e.g., sleep problems, irritability), and emotional numbing. Depression may be comorbid or secondary to PTSD. Alcohol or substance misuse may be a symptom or long-term complication. In the general population, the lifetime incidence of PTSD is 11.8%, compared to incidences between 3% and 58% in at-risk populations (such as combat veterans, natural disaster victims, victims of sexual assault). The *Impact of Event Scale-Revised* (IES-R) is an instrument to diagnose symptoms of PTSD. A cut-off of 33 for the total score has been found to provide best diagnostic criteria. Effective treatments include trauma-focused CBT and eye movement desensitization and reprocessing therapy (EMDR). Antidepressant drugs can be used as second-line treatment.

ASSESSMENT TIPS

Anxiety is a common symptom. Search for the specific diagnosis and possible psychiatric comorbidity.

Select specific psychometric tests to assess anxiety symptoms (e.g. panic, phobic, obsessive, post-traumatic) reported by the patient during the interview.

Investigate if the patient employs self-medication (anxiolytic and/or alcohol abuse) to cope with anxiety.

8.3   Bariatric Data

8.3.1   Anxiety Disorders

Compared to the general population, bariatric patients have a higher prevalence of anxiety disorders. Studies based on structured interviews (the best diagnostic method) have yielded variable prevalence rates. Malik et al. (2014) reported the lifetime and current prevalence rates of psychiatric disorders in 1089 bariatric surgery candidates diagnosed with structured interviews in five different studies. Current prevalence rates for anxiety disorders (including obsessive-compulsive disorder) ranged from 11.5 to 24%. Lifetime prevalence rates ranged from 15.5 to 37.5%. It is worth noting that the highest prevalence rates were found in the study of Kalarchian et al. (2007) where the evaluation process was independent of the approval process for the surgery (see below). Interviewing 393 Brazilian bariatric surgery candidates with the structured interview for DSM-IV diagnoses (SCID-I), Duarte-Guerra et al. (2015) reported a lifetime prevalence of anxiety disorders of 54.7% (current prevalence: 46.3%). The most common diagnosis was generalized anxiety disorder (current prevalence: 23.9%). A noteworthy finding of this study was the high rate of comorbidity of anxiety disorders with unipolar depression, bipolar disorder, and eating disorders.

In bariatric psychiatry, the reliability of prevalence data depends largely on the methodology of their collection. In some studies, the evaluation process was strictly independent of the approval process for the surgery and the participants were assured that information provided for research would not influence their eligibility for surgery. In other studies, the interviews were part of the pre-surgical evaluation interview, which might have led participants to selectively underreport some aspects of their psychiatric status or history in order to present themselves as psychologically healthy candidates. The studies with an independent evaluation process yielded results roughly comparable to each other and higher prevalence rates of psychiatric disorders than studies that did not have an independent assessment process. Thus, the prevalence rates of anxiety disorders in these studies may more accurately reflect the true prevalence of such problems. The difference between categorical diagnosis based on structured interviews and symptom rating based on questionnaires is another source of inconsistency. For example, Dawes et al. (2016) published a meta-analysis including 59 studies and 65,363 patients to determine the pre-operative point prevalence of mental health conditions among bariatric surgery candidates and recipients. Although the size of the meta-analysis in terms of both the number of studies included and patients enrolled makes the Dawes et al.'s study a landmark reference, the combination of diagnostic data based on either rating scales or structured interviews complicates the interpretation of the findings. Finally, attention should be paid to the specificity of diagnosis. For example, Fisher et al. (2017) conducted a large prospective (up to 2 years after surgery) study to compare bariatric surgery outcomes according to pre-operative psychiatric diagnosis. They combined patients with either depressive or anxiety disorders in a single diagnostic class subdivided on the basis of symptom severity (mild-to-moderate depression or anxiety and severe depression or anxiety).

In the light of these methodological problems, it is not surprising that data on both the post-operative course of anxiety and the impact of pre-operative anxiety on bariatric surgery outcome are inconsistent. The prospective study by de Zwaan et al. (2011) based on face-to-face (SCID-I) interviews found no significant decrease of the point prevalence of anxiety disorders after bariatric surgery: baseline, 16.8%; 6–12 months post-surgery, 15.3%; 24–36% months post-surgery, 14.3%. A recent systematic review assessed the short- (<24 months) and long-term (>24 months) effects of bariatric surgery on anxiety (Gill et al. 2019). Studies measuring anxiety with rating scales found small reductions in total anxiety scores with no major differences between the first 2 years after surgery and later post-surgery assessments. One study found increased levels of treatment for post-operative anxiety (Rutledge et al. 2012). Overall, these data confirm the clinical impression that, unlike depressive symptoms, anxiety symptoms do not improve substantially after bariatric surgery, not even when post-operative assessment is made in the short term.

de Zwaan et al. (2011) reported a differential effect of lifetime and current anxiety disorders on weight loss. Whereas current anxiety disorders had no impact, lifetime anxiety disorders were of negative prognostic value for post-operative weight loss. However, according to the majority of prospective studies, when successful outcome is measured in terms of weight loss, the impact of pre-operative anxiety seems to be negligible (Gill et al. 2019). Outcome measures other than weight loss offer a different perspective. Pre-operative anxiety correlates with post-operative anxiety and predicts an increased utilization of mental health services and poorer quality of life after surgery (Kalarchian et al. 2007; Morgan et al. 2019).

8.3.2 OCD

There are very few data on obsessive-compulsive disorder in bariatric patients. Both lifetime and current prevalence rates are relatively low and parallel those reported for the general population, which suggest that, in this regard, bariatric patients do not differ from other comparison groups. Kalarchian et al. (2007) reported a lifetime prevalence of 3.8% and a current prevalence of 2.1%. Likewise, in the study by Duarte-Guerra et al. (2015), the current prevalence was 3.6%. One exception is the study by Rutledge et al. (2011) on a cohort of surgery-eligible patients followed over time to assess how those pursuing bariatric surgery differed from those not pursuing or not approved for surgery. Bariatric patients reported higher rates of obsessive-compulsive disorder (28%) than the non-surgery patients (7%). The authors gave no explanation or interpretation for this unusual finding. No study reported on the post-surgery course of OCD or the prognostic value of OCD for surgery outcome.

8.3.3 PTSD

In the study of Duarte-Guerra et al. (2015), structured interviews of bariatric candidates gave a pre-operative prevalence rate of PTSD of 2.5%. After surgery, PTSD was the most persistent psychopathological condition. In the study of Walsh et al. (2017), of 3045 bariatric candidates, 216 (7.1%) had a diagnosis of current or past PTSD. Lifetime prevalence is around 11% (Kalarchian et al. 2007; Mitchell et al. 2012). Ikossi et al. (2010) conducted a study on 24 veterans with a diagnosis of PTSD who underwent gastric bypass. Their data suggested that bariatric surgery did not have a detrimental psychological effect on patients with PTSD, as only 2 of 24 patients demonstrated a worsening of symptoms at 12 months postoperatively. There was no significant difference between the percent excess weight lost after 1 year of follow-up between the PTSD group (66%) and the non-PTSD group (72%). Bariatric surgery had no beneficial effect on PTSD symptoms. Likewise, the bariatric patient with various psychiatric diagnoses including PTSD described in the case study of Peterhänsel et al. (2014) experienced no improvement in the post-traumatic symptoms after surgery. Based on the study of Sockalingam et al. (2013), PTSD is a predictor of non-completion of the pre-surgery assessment.

8.4 Clinical Management

According to the majority of studies, patients with anxiety disorders are eligible without question for bariatric surgery, need no specific interventions before surgery, and are expected to get post-surgery outcomes comparable to those of patients without anxiety disorders. Such an optimistic view is indirectly evidenced by the tendency to aggregate data on anxiety with those on depression, as if anxiety were a minor appendix to mood disorders.

Yet, data on anxiety disorders (and, by extension, on obsessive-compulsive disorder and post-traumatic stress disorder) in bariatric patients need to be qualified before translating them into the uncomplicated management strategies outlined above. We should evaluate cautiously the belief that these conditions are always benign and less relevant for bariatric surgery than disorders like eating disorders, depression, psychoses, and substance abuse.

First, their presumed low severity and modest disabling impact on daily life depends on the specific diagnosis. Unfortunately, such a specificity often got lost in most studies of bariatric patients. Specific phobias (e.g., fear of rats or darkness) are likely to have no relevance for admission to surgery and post-operative course. By contrast, severe forms obsessive-compulsive disorder and post-traumatic stress disorder can negatively impact several behaviors (e.g., coping with post-operative changes or modifying lifestyle habits) that are much relevant for bariatric surgery outcomes. The unwarranted emphasis on weight loss as the most important outcome has diverted clinicians' attention away from other variables that can jeopardize the mental well-being of bariatric patients with anxiety disorders. Second, many studies have aggregated data on anxiety with those on depression. The fact that the two conditions are often associated does not mean that they can be treated as different manifestations of the same syndrome. The post-operative course of anxiety is different from that of depression. After surgery, depression improves in the short term and sometimes recurs in the long term. By contrast, anxiety varies little over time and tends to persist. Third, anxiety disorders are highly comorbid with eating disorders, bipolar disorder, and substance abuse, and the presence of pathological anxiety is often a clue that should prompt the clinician to search for the symptoms of other psychiatric disorders.

In conclusion, to decide which is the best management of anxiety disorders in bariatric patients, we need more prospective studies enrolling patients with a specific diagnosis and no comorbidities; we need more prospective studies focusing on outcomes other than weight loss; and we need to know which is the prevalence of those patients' behaviors that are not listed among the symptoms of anxiety disorders but that are often induced by pathological anxiety (e.g., overuse of anxiolytic drugs in generalized anxiety disorder or alcohol use in post-traumatic stress disorder). Anxiety disorders are treatable, and, if the patient agrees, it is advisable to offer therapeutic interventions that can improve psychological well-being before surgery and optimize psychosocial outcomes after surgery.

KEY POINTS

Anxiety disorders are the most common mental disorders among patients seeking surgical treatment for obesity. Unlike OCD, PTSD has a high lifetime prevalence in bariatric candidates.

Pre-surgery anxiety correlates with post-surgery poorer quality of life, but it does not impact weight loss.

Anxiety symptoms do not improve after surgery.

References

Bandelow B, Reitt M, Röver C, Michaelis S, Görlich Y, Wedekind D. Efficacy of treatments for anxiety disorders: a meta-analysis. Int Clin Psychopharmacol. 2015;30(4):183–92. Review. PubMed PMID: 25932596. https://doi.org/10.1097/YIC.0000000000000078.

Dawes AJ, Maggard-Gibbons M, Maher AR, Booth MJ, Miake-Lye I, Beroes JM, Shekelle PG. Mental health conditions among patients seeking and undergoing bariatric surgery: a meta-analysis. JAMA. 2016;315(2):150–63. PubMed PMID: 26757464. https://doi.org/10.1001/jama.2015.18118.

de Zwaan M, Enderle J, Wagner S, Mühlhans B, Ditzen B, Gefeller O, Mitchell JE, Müller A. Anxiety and depression in bariatric surgery patients: a prospective, follow-up study using structured clinical interviews. J Affect Disord. 2011;133(1–2):61–8. Epub 2011 Apr 17. PubMed PMID: 21501874. https://doi.org/10.1016/j.jad.2011.03.025.

Duarte-Guerra LS, Coêlho BM, Santo MA, Wang YP. Psychiatric disorders among obese patients seeking bariatric surgery: results of structured clinical interviews. Obes Surg. 2015;25(5):830–7. PubMed PMID: 25358821. https://doi.org/10.1007/s11695-014-1464-y.

Fisher D, Coleman KJ, Arterburn DE, Fischer H, Yamamoto A, Young DR, Sherwood NE, Trinacty CM, Lewis KH. Mental illness in bariatric surgery: a cohort study from the PORTAL network. Obesity (Silver Spring). 2017;25(5):850–6. PubMed PMID: 28440047. https://doi.org/10.1002/oby.21814.

Gill H, Kang S, Lee Y, Rosenblat JD, Brietzke E, Zuckerman H, McIntyre RS. The long-term effect of bariatric surgery on depression and anxiety. J Affect Disord. 2019;246:886–94. Epub 2018 Dec 28. PubMed PMID: 30795495. https://doi.org/10.1016/j.jad.2018.12.113.

Ikossi DG, Maldonado JR, Hernandez-Boussard T, Eisenberg D. Post-traumatic stress disorder (PTSD) is not a contraindication to gastric bypass in veterans with morbid obesity. Surg Endosc. 2010;24(8):1892–7. Epub 2010 Jan 9. PubMed PMID: 20063014. https://doi.org/10.1007/s00464-009-0866-8.

Kalarchian MA, Marcus MD, Levine MD, Courcoulas AP, Pilkonis PA, Ringham RM, Soulakova JN, Weissfeld LA, Rofey DL. Psychiatric disorders among bariatric surgery candidates: relationship to obesity and functional health status. Am J Psychiatry. 2007;164(2):328–34; quiz 374. PubMed PMID: 17267797.

Malik S, Mitchell JE, Engel S, Crosby R, Wonderlich S. Psychopathology in bariatric surgery candidates: a review of studies using structured diagnostic interviews. Compr Psychiatry. 2014;55(2):248–59. Epub 2013 Oct 24. Review. PubMed PMID: 24290079; PubMed Central PMCID: PMC3985130. https://doi.org/10.1016/j.comppsych.2013.08.021.

Mitchell JE, Selzer F, Kalarchian MA, Devlin MJ, Strain GW, Elder KA, Marcus MD, Wonderlich S, Christian NJ, Yanovski SZ. Psychopathology before surgery in the longitudinal assessment of bariatric surgery-3 (LABS-3) psychosocial study. Surg Obes Relat Dis. 2012;8(5):533–41. Epub 2012 Jul 14. PubMed PMID: 22920965; PubMed Central PMCID: PMC3584713. https://doi.org/10.1016/j.soard.2012.07.001.

Morgan DJR, Ho KM, Platell C. Incidence and determinants of mental health service use after bariatric surgery. JAMA Psychiat. 2019. [Epub ahead of print] PubMed PMID: 31553420; PubMed Central PMCID: PMC6763981. https://doi.org/10.1001/jamapsychiatry.2019.2741.

Peterhänsel C, Wagner B, Dietrich A, Kersting A. Obesity and co-morbid psychiatric disorders as contraindications for bariatric surgery? A case study. Int J Surg Case Rep. 2014;5(12):1268–70. Epub 2014 Nov 13. PubMed PMID: 25460490; PubMed Central PMCID: PMC4275787. https://doi.org/10.1016/j.ijscr.2014.11.023.

Rutledge T, Adler S, Friedman R. A prospective assessment of psychosocial factors among bariatric versus non-bariatric surgery candidates. Obes Surg. 2011;21(10):1570–9. PubMed PMID: 20872090; PubMed Central PMCID: PMC3179584. https://doi.org/10.1007/s11695-010-0287-8.

Rutledge T, Braden AL, Woods G, Herbst KL, Groesz LM, Savu M. Five-year changes in psychiatric treatment status and weight-related comorbidities following bariatric surgery in a veteran population. Obes Surg. 2012;22(11):1734–41. PubMed PMID: 23011461. https://doi.org/10.1007/s11695-012-0722-0.

Sockalingam S, Cassin S, Crawford SA, Pitzul K, Khan A, Hawa R, Jackson T, Okrainec A. Psychiatric predictors of surgery non-completion following suitability assessment for bariatric surgery. Obes Surg. 2013;23(2):205–11. PubMed PMID: 22961685. https://doi.org/10.1007/s11695-012-0762-5.

Walsh E, Rosenstein L, Dalrymple K, Chelminski I, Zimmerman M. The importance of assessing for childhood abuse and lifetime PTSD in bariatric surgery candidates. J Clin Psychol Med Settings. 2017;24(3-4):341–54. PubMed PMID: 29159539. https://doi.org/10.1007/s10880-017-9518-7.

Personality Disorders

9

Abstract

An increasing degree of severity of obesity is accompanied by a rising prevalence of personality disorders, reaching 23.4% for obesity class III. Yet, there are
few studies that have focused on the relationship between bariatric surgery and
personality disorders. Preliminary data show that personality disorders do not
impact weight loss but weight loss seems to influence the course of personality
disorders. Four independent studies assessing bariatric surgery in a total of 570
patients found that there was no significant predictive value of a personality disorder in terms of post-operative weight loss. One study investigated whether the
course of personality disorders was influenced by massive weight loss in the first
year after bariatric surgery. There was a significant reduction in the prevalence of
personality disorders from 22 to 8% at 1-year follow-up. This was particularly
evident for avoidant personality disorder. A possible explanation is that post-
surgery weight loss reduces social stigmatization associated with severe obesity.
While taking care of bariatric patients with personality disorders, the clinician
should focus on two aspects: (1) the behaviors caused by the personality disorder
that interfere with pre- and post-operative programs and (2) the interpersonal
problems caused by the personality disorder that threaten the development of an
optimal therapeutic relationship.

Keywords

Personality disorders · Screening questionnaires · Structured interview
Interpersonal behavior · Therapeutic relationship

© Springer Nature Switzerland AG 2020
A. Troisi, *Bariatric Psychology and Psychiatry*,
https://doi.org/10.1007/978-3-030-44834-9_9

9.1   Background

In their comprehensive review of the relationship between obesity and personality disorders, Gerlach et al. (2016) concluded that an increasing degree of severity of obesity is accompanied by a rising prevalence of personality disorders, reaching 23.4% for obesity class III. Based on these data (that emerged from a total of 68 studies), we could expect that personality disorders have been largely studied in bariatric patients. Unfortunately, this is not the case. There are few studies that have focused on the relationship between bariatric surgery and personality disorders, and some of them have a methodological quality that questions the validity of their findings.

This chapter outlines the classification and clinical features of personality disorders, explains how to obtain diagnostic information, reports data on their prevalence in bariatric patients, and analyzes various aspects of their interface with bariatric surgery (i.e., impact of personality disorders on post-surgery outcome, impact of bariatric surgery on the course of personality disorders, and the pre- and postoperative clinical management of personality disorders).

9.2   Basic Notions

Personality disorders are deeply ingrained and enduring patterns of inner experience and behavior that deviate markedly from expectations in the individual's culture, lead to subjective distress and sometimes cause others distress, and are relatively pervasive and inflexible. Personality disorders normally start in childhood or adolescence. In the adult population, personality disorders of at least mild severity have a prevalence ranging between 4 and 13%. In psychiatric outpatients, prevalence is much higher and reach 30%.

DSM-5 lists ten specific personality disorders that are grouped in three clusters based on descriptive similarities. Cluster A (odd) includes three personality disorders (paranoid, schizoid, schizotypal) that are related to psychotic disorders with the important difference that hallucinations and true delusions are absent. Cluster B (dramatic) includes four personality disorders (antisocial, borderline, histrionic, narcissistic) that are characterized by emotional instability and manipulative behaviors. Cluster C (fearful) includes three personality disorders (avoidant, dependent, and obsessive-compulsive) that have, in common, exaggerated fears and negative affectivity. One of the key changes from DSM-IV to DSM-5 was the elimination of the multiaxial system including Axis II that was reserved for personality disorders and mental retardation. Yet, common clinical language still uses the expression "Axis II disorders" as a synonymous for personality disorders.

Personality disorders are complex and difficult to diagnose. Even when a personality disorder is identified, significant comorbidities often go undetected. Patients often need support that goes beyond healthcare, and this makes care planning complex. Carrying out a structured assessment using recognized tools is essential to identify a range of symptoms, make an accurate diagnosis, and recognize comorbidities. The *Structured Clinical Interview for DSM-5 Personality Disorders* (SCID-5-PD) is used to evaluate the 10 DSM-5 personality disorders. The SCID-5-PD name reflects the elimination of the multiaxial system in DSM-5. Although the DSM-IV personality disorder criteria are unchanged in DSM-5, the SCID-5-PD interview questions have been thoroughly reviewed and revised to optimally capture the construct embodied in the diagnostic criteria.

To save time, screening questionnaires can be administered before deciding if a structured interview is necessary or not. The *Personality Disorders Questionnaire* (PDQ-IV) is a 99-item self-report measure used to identify the key features or possible presence of a personality disorder. The PDQ-IV uses one question (e.g., *Some people think I take advantage of others.*) to assess each specific DSM-IV personality criterion (e.g., narcissistic personality disorder: lacks empathy), and responses are in a true/false format, with the exception of the last two items, which are checklists of behaviors. The *Millon Clinical Multiaxial Inventory, 3rd edition* (MCMI-III) is composed of 175 true-false questions and usually takes the average person less than 30 min to complete. After the test is scored, it produces 28 scales: 24 personality and clinical scales and 4 scales used to verify how the person approached and took the test. It is shorter than other personality tests, such as the MMPI-2 which has 567 true/false questions. It can be administered and scored on the computer in a psychologist's office. The MCMI-III is coordinated to the DSM-IV personality disorders and other major clinical diagnoses.

Because the cognitive, emotional, and behavioral traits of personality disorders tend to be stable over time, these disorders have been considered not amenable to treatment. However, multiple treatments are now available, including interpersonal psychotherapy, cognitive behavior therapy, dialectical behavior therapy, mentalization-based therapy, and pharmacotherapy (e.g., typical and atypical antipsychotics, antidepressants, mood stabilizers). Although these treatments have been studied for use in several personality disorders, most of the medical literature is limited to borderline personality disorder. In patients with avoidant personality disorder and comorbid binge eating, Robinson and Safer (2012) have shown the utility of a modified version of dialectical behavior therapy (DBT-BED) aiming at an enhancement of emotion regulation capacities. Similar findings have reported in bariatric patients with comorbid borderline personality disorder and bulimia nervosa (Gallé et al. 2017).

Assessment tips
Personality disorders are complex and difficult to diagnose.
Even when a personality disorder is identified, significant comorbidities often go undetected.
Carrying out a structured assessment using recognized tools is essential to identify a range of symptoms, make an accurate diagnosis, and recognize comorbidities.
To save time, screening questionnaires (PDQ-IV, MCMI-III) can be administered before deciding if a structured interview is necessary or not.

9.3   Bariatric Data

In the sample of 288 bariatric candidates studied by Kalarchian et al. (2007), the total prevalence of personality disorders was 28.5%, with avoidant personality disorder being the most common specific diagnosis (17%). Compared to other studies, the validity and reliability of these findings are excellent for two reasons. First, the evaluation process was strictly independent of the approval process for the surgery and the participants were assured that information provided for research would not influence their eligibility for surgery. Second, diagnosis was based on a structured interview specifically designed for the identification of DSM personality disorders (SCID-II). In the Italian study by Mauri et al. (2008), the most common Axis II was obsessive-compulsive personality disorder (13.9% of 282 participants). Malik et al. (2014) suggested two possible interpretations for the finding that in both studies the most prevalent personality disorders belonged to Cluster C. It is possible that social stigma, discrimination, and fears of negative social evaluation may exacerbate anxious or avoidant traits in extremely obese individuals, which might result in higher rates of Cluster C personality disorders. An alternative possibility is that avoidant and obsessive-compulsive personality disorder may result in a greater likelihood of engaging in disordered eating behavior leading to obesity.

The widely different prevalence rates reported by other studies invite reflections on the methods for diagnosing personality disorders in bariatric patients. For example, the meta-analysis of mental health conditions among bariatric patients published by Dawes et al. (2016) reported a pre-operative prevalence rate of about 6% (184 patients with personality disorders out of 3002 patients reporting data). By contrast, the review by Gerlach et al. (2016) reported much higher prevalence rates for any personality disorder: an average prevalence of 24.5% in interview-based studies and an average prevalence of 37.2% in questionnaire-based studies. Even if the discrepancy between data based on interviews and those based on questionnaires partly explains inconsistent findings, other factors are likely to be involved. For example, the prevalence of borderline personality disorder was 0% in two different studies, one based on interviews (Pontiroli et al. 2007) and the other on questionnaires (Martínez et al. 2013). It is likely that some bariatric candidates avoid reporting dysfunctional emotions and behaviors lest to be denied surgery.

Data on post-surgery outcome are consistent. All four studies assessing bariatric surgery in a total of 570 patients (Black et al. 2003; Grana et al. 1989; Kalarchian et al. 2008; Pontiroli et al. 2007) found that there was no significant predictive value of a personality disorder in terms of post-operative weight loss. The observation periods in these studies lie between 6 months and 4 years. The personality disorder spectrum in the various studies differed clearly, consisting partly of predominantly Cluster A personality disorders (49%), partly of narcissistic personality disorders (6.9%) and partly of avoidant personality disorders (8.6%). Based on these findings, Gerlach et al. (2016) concluded that a pre-operatively diagnosed personality disorder did not have a significant influence on post-operative weight loss. However, in view of the short follow-up periods, the post-operative effects can only be interpreted with caution.

Personality disorders do not impact weight loss, but weight loss seems to influence the course of personality disorders. Lier et al. (2013) investigated whether the course of personality disorders is influenced by massive weight loss in the first year after bariatric surgery. They observed a significant reduction in the prevalence of personality disorders from 22% to 8% at 1-year follow-up. This was particularly evident for avoidant personality disorder. A possible explanation is that post-surgery weight loss reduces social stigmatization associated with severe obesity, and such an improvement in social interactions may decrease patients' anxious preoccupation with the fear of negative evaluation and rejection.

9.4   Clinical Management

Patients with personality disorders seek psychiatric evaluation and treatment less often than patients with other mental disorders. When they seek help, often they are motivated by symptoms of comorbid psychopathology that mask the primary personality disorder. In addition, the major impact of personality disorders on interpersonal functioning can complicate the therapeutic relationship. All these reasons make clinical management of personality disorders very difficult. This is also certainly true for bariatric patients with a diagnosis of personality disorder. While taking care of these patients, the clinician should focus on two aspects: (1) the behaviors caused by the personality disorder that interfere with pre- and post-operative programs and (2) the interpersonal problems caused by the personality disorder that threaten the development of an optimal therapeutic relationship.

Dysfunctional behaviors associated with pathological personality often present as symptoms of other mental disorders, and this makes their identification and treatment more difficult. For example, a patient with borderline personality disorder can present with binge eating and alcohol abuse. These disordered behaviors originate from the combination of trait impulsivity with episodic dysphoria, which are typical features of borderline personality disorder. The patient is unable to cope with negative emotions and resorts impulsively to compensatory rewards. Binge eating and alcohol abuse can be isolated symptoms or exceed the threshold for the diagnosis of comorbid conditions. In either case, short-term treatment and prevention should target the dysfunctional behaviors as in primary binge eating disorder or substance misuse. Yet, the presence of an underlying borderline personality disorder needs to be detected because it may require more comprehensive intervention strategies (e.g., psychotherapy focusing on emotion regulation) (Gerlach et al. 2016).

Working with patients with personality disorders (especially those with Cluster A and B personality disorders) is difficult and requires specific training. Forming a therapeutic alliance is problematic with patients who have distorted core beliefs of others that lead them to enact dysfunctional interpersonal behaviors (Table 9.1). Each member of the multidisciplinary team taking pre- and post-operative care of bariatric patients should be aware of such potential difficulties.

Table 9.1 Possible impact of personality disorders on therapeutic relationship and post-operative behavior

PERSONALITY DISORDER	THERAPEUTIC RELATIONSHIP	POST-OPERATIVE BEHAVIOR
SCHIZOID	Difficulty establishing and maintaining a therapeutic relationship.	Missing follow-up appointments.
SCHIZOTYPICAL	Ideas of reference about clinical prescriptions.	Idiosyncratic implementation of post-operative program.
PARANOID	Doubting every guidance provided by the clinician.	Accusations and potentially litigious threats from the patient.
BORDERLINE	Alternating between extremes of idealization and devaluation.	Impulsive behaviors including disordered eating.
HISTRIONIC	Excessive attention seeking.	Dramatic reporting of physical symptoms.
ANTISOCIAL	Failure to conform to social norms regulating doctor–patient relationship.	Manipulative and/or hostile attitude toward the clinician.
NARCISSISTIC	Unreasonable expectations of especially favorable treatment.	Unfounded claims of medical negligence.
AVOIDANT	Inhibition of open communication because of fear of being criticized.	Failure to report relevant clinical information.
OBSESSIVE-COMPULSIVE	Preoccupations with details of clinical indications at the expense of effective collaboration.	Repeated request for the explanation of irrelevant technical details.
DEPENDENT	Excessive need to be taken care of.	Request for extra follow-up appointments.

KEY POINTS

Prevalence of personality disorders is high among bariatric patients.

Personality disorders do not impact weight loss, but weight loss seems to influence the course of personality disorders.

Clinical management should target: (1) the behaviors that interfere with pre- and post-operative programs and (2) the interpersonal problems that threaten the development of an optimal therapeutic relationship.

References

Black DW, Goldstein RB, Mason EE. Psychiatric diagnosis and weight loss following gastric surgery for obesity. Obes Surg. 2003;13:746–51.

Dawes AJ, Maggard-Gibbons M, Maher AR, Booth MJ, Miake-Lye I, Beroes JM, Shekelle PG. Mental health conditions among patients seeking and undergoing bariatric surgery: a meta-analysis. JAMA. 2016;315(2):150–63. PubMed PMID: 26757464. https://doi.org/10.1001/jama.2015.18118.

Gallé F, Maida P, Cirella A, Giuliano E, Belfiore P, Liguori G. Does post-operative psychotherapy contribute to improved comorbidities in bariatric patients with borderline personality disorder traits and bulimia tendencies? A prospective study. Obes Surg. 2017;27(7):1872–8. PubMed PMID: 28181141. https://doi.org/10.1007/s11695-017-2581-1.

Gerlach G, Loeber S, Herpertz S. Personality disorders and obesity: a systematic review. Obes Rev. 2016;17(8):691–723. Epub 2016 May 27. Review. PubMed PMID: 27230851. https://doi.org/10.1111/obr.12415.

Grana AS, Coolidge FL, Merwin MM. Personality profiles of the morbidly obese. J Clin Psychol. 1989;45:762–5.

Kalarchian MA, Marcus MD, Levine MD, Courcoulas AP, Pilkonis PA, Ringham RM, Soulakova JN, Weissfeld LA, Rofey DL. Psychiatric disorders among bariatric surgery candidates: relationship to obesity and functional health status. Am J Psychiatry. 2007;164(2):328–34; quiz 374. PubMed PMID: 17267797.

Kalarchian MA, Marcus MD, Levine MD, Soulakova JN, Courcoulas AP, Wisinski MS. Relationship of psychiatric disorders to 6-month outcomes after gastric bypass. Surg Obes Relat Dis. 2008;4:544–9.

Lier HØ, Biringer E, Stubhaug B, Tangen T. Prevalence of psychiatric disorders before and 1 year after bariatric surgery: the role of shame in maintenance of psychiatric disorders in patients undergoing bariatric surgery. Nord J Psychiatry. 2013;67(2):89–96. Epub 2012 May 16. PubMed PMID: 22587601. https://doi.org/10.3109/08039488.2012.684703.

Malik S, Mitchell JE, Engel S, Crosby R, Wonderlich S. Psychopathology in bariatric surgery candidates: a review of studies using structured diagnostic interviews. Compr Psychiatry. 2014;55(2):248–59. Epub 2013 Oct 24. Review. PubMed PMID: 24290079; PubMed Central PMCID: PMC3985130. https://doi.org/10.1016/j.comppsych.2013.08.021.

Martínez EP, González ST, Vicente MM, van der Hofstadt Román CJ, Rodríguez-Marín J. Psychopathology in a sample of candidate patients for bariatric surgery. Int J Psychiatry Clin Pract. 2013;17(3):197–205. Epub 2012 Jul 21. PubMed PMID: 22746988. https://doi.org/10.3109/13651501.2012.704383.

Mauri M, Rucci P, Calderone A, Santini F, Oppo A, Romano A, Rinaldi S, Armani A, Polini M, Pinchera A, Cassano GB. Axis I and II disorders and quality of life in bariatric surgery candidates. J Clin Psychiatry. 2008;69(2):295–301. PubMed PMID: 18251626.

Pontiroli AE, Fossati A, Vedani P. Post-surgery adherence to scheduled visits and compliance, more than personality disorders, predict outcome of bariatric restrictive surgery in morbidly obese patients. Obes Surg. 2007;17:1492–7.

Robinson AH, Safer DL. Moderators of dialectical behavior therapy for binge eating disorder: results from a randomized controlled trial. Int J Eat Disord. 2012;45(4):597–602. Epub 2011 Apr 15. PubMed PMID: 21500238; PubMed Central PMCID: PMC3155005. https://doi.org/10.1002/eat.20932.

Bipolar Disorder

10

Abstract

Bariatric candidates presenting with depressive symptoms represent a challenge for differential diagnosis. A patient may present with the classic symptoms of depression but may actually be suffering from bipolar disorder. It is very important to avoid the trap of diagnosing depressive disorder too quickly and to consider all the clinical aspects that can instead suggest bipolar disorder. The evidence thus far suggests that surgery is likely a safe option for patients with well-controlled bipolar disorder. Yet, unstable symptomatic bipolar disorder is an absolute contraindication for bariatric surgery. Lithium remains the best established long-term treatment for bipolar disorder. Given its narrow therapeutic index and potential for toxicity, lithium treatment requires special care in the perioperative period. The main goals of adjunctive psychotherapy for bipolar disorder include the education of patients, and when possible, caregivers, strategies for the management of stress, the identification and intervention of early signs of recurrence, the enhancement of adherence with drug regimens, and how to keep regular lifestyle habits (e.g., regular sleep pattern and healthy nutrition).

Keywords

Bipolar disorder · Bipolar depression · Psychiatric contraindication · Lithium toxicity · Adjunctive psychotherapy

10.1 Background

Bipolar disorder includes a range of illnesses in which there are disturbances of mood into both depression and elation, i.e., the poles of affective experience. Numerous studies show that patients with bipolar disorder are at an increased risk for overweight and obesity (Reilly-Harrington et al. 2018). For example,

© Springer Nature Switzerland AG 2020
A. Troisi, *Bariatric Psychology and Psychiatry*,
https://doi.org/10.1007/978-3-030-44834-9_10

researchers from Spain analyzed the data of 86,028 patients in a Health Management Organization and found that patients with bipolar disorder showed a significantly higher frequency of obesity (41%) than those patients without bipolar disorder (27%) (Sicras et al. 2008).

Several factors can explain the high prevalence of obesity among bipolar patients. Many medication treatments for bipolar disorder are associated with weight gain, including lithium and valproic acid among traditional mood stabilizers, and most second-generation antipsychotics that are being increasingly used in the acute and maintenance treatment of bipolar disorder. Although medications often play a significant role in weight gain, there is evidence that the prevalence of obesity is also higher among untreated bipolar patients. These observational data suggest the existence of pleiotropic genes and biological pathways shared by bipolar disorder and cardiometabolic diseases (Amare et al. 2017). Another potential contributing factor to obesity in bipolar disorder is the frequent comorbidity with eating disorders. The presence of binge eating disorder comorbid with bipolar disorder has been associated with obesity and cardiovascular disease, as well as greater mood instability, residual mood symptoms, psychosis, anxiety, and suicidality (Boulanger et al. 2018).

Given the high rate of overlap between bipolar disorder and obesity, it is not surprising that patients with bipolar disorder seek surgical options for obesity treatment. This chapter outlines basic notions on bipolar disorder; reviews published data on the indications, contraindications, and outcomes of bariatric surgery in patients with bipolar disorder; and illustrates assessment procedures that can inform the clinical decision to offer or not surgical treatment to this patient population.

10.2 Basic Notions

The cardinal clinical feature of bipolar disorder is the presence of at least one episode of mania or hypomania. Current classification systems distinguish between bipolar I disorder (one or more manic or mixed episodes and usually one or more major depressive episodes), bipolar II disorder (recurrent major depressive and hypomanic but not manic episodes), and cyclothymic disorder (chronic mood fluctuations over at least 2 years, with episodes of depression and hypomania of insufficient severity to meet the diagnostic criteria for bipolar II disorder). The difference between hypomania and mania lies in the severity of symptoms (Table 10.1). Severe episodes of mania can be complicated by psychotic symptoms (delusions and/or hallucinations).

The depressive episodes seen in bipolar disorder are very like other types of depressive illness. On average, marked slowing of thought and action is more common in bipolar than in unipolar patients. Psychotic depression in younger people and atypical features of depression, such as hypersomnia, are also more common. In a patient with major depression, a first-degree relative with bipolar disorder may also suggest a bipolar diagnosis.

Lifetime prevalence is 1% for bipolar I disorder, 0.4–2% for bipolar II disorder, and 2.5% for cyclothymic disorder. The female/male ratio is approximately equal

Table 10.1 Symptoms of mania (severe) or hypomania (mild)

SYMPTOM
Elation
Irritability
Increased energy
Decreased need for sleep
Grandiosity
Increased amount and speed of speech
Increased sexual drive
Racing thoughts
Poor judgement in relation money, sex, and driving
Inappropriate social behavior

for bipolar I disorder. Some but not all studies show a female excess in the bipolar II group. Peak age of onset is in the early twenties. Bipolar disorder tends to persist life-long, but its course is very variable. Depression is usually the predominant abnormality of mood and an important cause of functional impairment in bipolar patients and contributes to their increased mortality from suicide. There is an overall increase in premature mortality, only partially explained by a suicide rate of 10%. Prognosis for bipolar II disorder is better, although there remains a high suicide risk.

10.3 Assessment

The diagnosis of bipolar disorder is easy if the patient is examined during a manic or hypomanic episode and when the patient reports a personal history of mania or hypomania. Yet, in the following cases, the diagnosis is difficult: (1) the patient is symptom-free and does not report previous episodes of mania or hypomania; (2) the patient presents with depressive symptoms and does not report previous episodes of mania or hypomania.

Patients may not initially reveal to the clinician that they have previously had a manic or hypomanic episode. Thus, it is very important to ask specific questions that unmask symptoms suggesting a diagnosis of bipolar disorder. All the relevant questions are included in a brief self-report instrument (the *Mood Disorder Questionnaire,* MDQ) that takes about 5 min to complete. The MDQ is designed for screening purposes only and is not to be used as a diagnostic tool. A positive screen should be followed by a comprehensive evaluation. The MDQ is best at screening for bipolar I disorder and is less sensitive to bipolar II disorder or bipolar not otherwise specified disorder. The MDQ includes 13 questions (e.g., "Has there ever been a period of time when you were not your usual self and you felt much more self-confident than usual?" "Has there ever been a period of time when you were not your usual self and you were more talkative or spoke much faster than usual?" "Has there ever been a period of time when you were not your usual self and you had more energy than usual?"). In order to screen positive, the patient should answer "yes" to 7 or more of the 13 items.

Bariatric candidates presenting with depressive symptoms represent a challenge for differential diagnosis. Throughout the course of bipolar disorder, depressive episodes are generally more frequent than manic or hypomanic episodes. A patient may present with the classic symptoms of depression but may actually be suffering from bipolar disorder. It is very important to avoid the trap of diagnosing depressive disorder too quickly and to consider all the clinical aspects that can instead suggest bipolar disorder. Compared to unipolar depression, bipolar depression is often associated with distinctive clinical features that can lead to the right diagnosis (Table 10.2). Yet, it is worth noting that none of these clinical features is pathognomonic. Only previous episodes of mania or hypomania make the diagnosis of bipolar disorder certain.

Once a diagnosis of bipolar disorder has been formulated, the next step is to ascertain if the patient is currently symptomatic or not. Complete remission requires the absence of clinically relevant symptoms. The *Young Mania Rating Scale* (YMRS) is

Table 10.2 Clues that may differentiate bipolar (BD) from unipolar major depression (MD)

CLINICAL FEATURE	BD vs. MD
Family history of bipolar disorder	BD > MD
Earlier age of onset	BD > MD
Anergia	BD > MD
Hypersomnolence	BD > MD
Hyperphagia	BD > MD
Psychomotor retardation	BD > MD
Irritability	BD > MD
Racing thoughts	BD > MD
Anticipatory anhedonia	BD > MD
Tearfulness	MD > BD
Anxiety	MD > BD
Tendency to blame others	MD > BD
Initial insomnia	MD > BD

one of the most frequently utilized rating scales to assess manic symptoms. The scale has 11 items and is based on the patient's subjective report of his or her clinical condition over the previous 48 h. Additional information is based upon clinical observations made during the course of the clinical interview. The items are selected based upon published descriptions of the core symptoms of mania. There are four items that are graded on a 0–8 scale (irritability, speech, thought content, and disruptive/aggressive behavior), while the remaining seven items are graded on a 0–4 scale. These four items are given twice the weight of the others to compensate for poor cooperation from severely ill patients. There are well-described anchor points for each grade of severity. Strengths of the YMRS include its brevity, widely accepted use, and ease of administration. The scale is generally done by a clinician or other trained rater with expertise with manic patients and takes 15–30 min to complete.

The administration of the YMRS should be integrated by assessing the presence and severity of depressive symptoms with a depression rating scale. There are many questionnaires that can be used for the screening of depression, including the *Beck Depression Inventory* (BDI), the *Patient Health Questionnaire-9* (PHQ-9), the *Montgomery-Åsberg Depression Rating Scale* (MADRS), and the *Hamilton Depression Rating Scale* (HDRS).

A crucial aspect of assessment is the diagnostic search for comorbid psychopathology. Bipolar disorder is highly comorbid with other psychiatric disorders including eating disorders, substance use disorders, and borderline personality disorder. Missing the diagnosis of comorbid disorders jeopardizes the validity and utility of pre-surgery mental assessment and increases the risk of poor outcome.

Assessment tips
The diagnosis of bipolar disorder is difficult when the patient does not report previous episodes of mania or hypomania and is symptom-free or presents with depressive symptoms.
The MDQ is a useful screening test to unmask symptoms suggesting a diagnosis of bipolar disorder.
The YMRS measures the presence and severity of manic symptoms.
Patients with bipolar disorder need post-operative long-term assessment.

10.4   Bariatric Data

Clinical research on weight loss and psychiatric outcomes in patients with bipolar disorder who underwent bariatric surgery is based on limited evidence. In addition, the studies with the largest samples failed to distinguish bipolar patients from psychiatric patients with other severe mental disorders. These methodological aspects complicate the interpretation of findings.

To compare bariatric surgery (vertical sleeve gastrectomy or Roux-en-Y gastric bypass) outcomes according to preoperative mental illness category, Fisher et al.

(2017) published a large retrospective cohort study including 8192 patients with a mean post-operative enrollment span of 2.9 years. The sample included 508 patients with a diagnosis of bipolar disorder, psychosis, or schizophrenia. Their weight loss was very similar to that recorded in patients with no pre-operative mental illness. However, the subgroup of patients with severe mental illness had a greater acute care use (i.e., emergency department visits and hospital days) beginning as soon as 3 months after surgery and persisting through 2 years of follow-up.

Kouidrat et al. (2017) published a systematic review of the outcomes of bariatric surgery among patients with severe mental disorders (i.e., bipolar disorder or schizophrenia). The review was based on eight studies including a total of 279 participants. The mean length of follow-up was 15.7 months (range 12 to 24). Of the eight studies, two were prospective cohort studies and six involved a control group of participants without a psychiatric diagnosis. Regarding specifically bipolar patients, results of six studies ($N = 121$) showed a significant mean excess weight loss (%EWL) from baseline to 24 months, ranging from −31 to −70%. One study examined weight change occurring greater than 24 months after surgery and found no differences in weight between patients with bipolar disorder and matched control patients who attended medical follow-up care at 24 months or longer (average of 52 months) after surgery.

Steinmann et al. (2011) compared 33 patients with bipolar disorder to patients matched by age and gender with another psychiatric disorder or with no psychiatric disorder. They found lower starting BMIs in the non-psychiatric group compared to the other groups, but no differences in weight loss at 6 and 12 months. A large study compared 144 bipolar patients who underwent bariatric surgery with 1440 matched unexposed controls who were followed for a mean of 2 years. The surgical intervention was not associated with significant differences in the risk of psychiatric hospitalization or change in rate of outpatient visits for psychiatric services (Ahmed et al. 2013). A retrospective database study compared bariatric candidates who were diagnosed with bipolar disorder to matched controls without bipolar disorder. Authors looked at weight loss over a follow-up that ranged from 3 to 10 years and found similar weight losses between groups among those who went on to have surgery. They did find that patients with bipolar disorder were less likely to attend follow-up appointments two or more years after surgery than those without bipolar disorder (Friedman et al. 2017).

Data on pre-operative selection are useful to put the findings on weight loss and psychiatric outcomes into the right perspective. Some candidate patients with bipolar disorder may be prevented from having surgery because of their clinical profiles. It is possible that these patients would have worse post-surgery outcomes and that the findings of the studies discussed above reflect a positive bias due to pre-operative selection.

Grothe et al. (2014) have examined rates of surgical recommendation among patients with bipolar disorder. Among 935 patients who had a pre-surgical psychological evaluation, 6% screened positive for symptoms of bipolar disorder. For 13% of this group, it was decided that surgery was not an appropriate treatment option for psychiatric reasons, and yet only 22% of patients with bipolar disorder went on to have surgery (compared to 34% of patients seeking surgery without bipolar disorder). Patients with bipolar disorder who did have surgery reported better baseline mental health than those who did not have surgery, specifically endorsing lower anxiety, lower emotional and physical neglect, higher distress tolerance, and more confidence in controlling eating. In the study by Friedman et al. (2017), pre-surgical screening identified 73 patients with bipolar disorder out of 3263 bariatric candidates. Of these, 36% were initially recommended for surgery, 45% were initially delayed for surgery, and 19% were initially informed that surgery was not recommended. In total, 48% of individuals seeking surgery with bipolar disorder ultimately had surgery and 52% did not. Patients without a history of psychiatric hospitalization were more likely to be recommended for surgery.

Based on these data, it is clear that a substantial number of patients with bipolar disorder are prevented from having bariatric surgery for psychiatric reasons. Reilly-Harrington et al. (2018) have suggested that stigma may play a role in the lower rates of recommendations for surgery among patients with serious mental illness (e.g., the belief that those with mental illness are irresponsible and their life decisions should be made by others). They have argued that surgical recommendations should be based on more research into adherence to surgery-specific behaviors postoperatively along with improved training into the management of severe mental illness in the surgery setting.

10.5   Clinical Management

Bipolar disorder is a life-long illness that requires long-term monitoring and maintenance treatment. After initial onset, patients with bipolar disorder have residual depressive symptoms for about a third of the weeks of their lives. Patients also experience psychotic symptoms, impaired functioning, compromised quality of life, and stigma. Even with treatment, about 37% of patients relapse into depression or mania within 1 year, and 60% within 2 years. Based on these data, it is evident that patients who go on to have bariatric surgery need careful perioperative and postoperative management (Shelby et al. 2015; Taylor and Misra 2009). Management should focus on the optimization of pharmacotherapy and the implementation of psychosocial support.

Lithium remains the best established long-term treatment for bipolar disorder. It is readily and completely absorbed in the small intestine. Lithium is hydrophilic and nonprotein bound, is not metabolized, and is almost completely excreted by the kidney. Given its narrow therapeutic index and potential for toxicity, lithium treatment requires special care in the perioperative period because of changes in oral intake and fluid and electrolyte shifts. Toxicity is the immediate concern for bariatric patients on lithium treatment (Alam et al. 2016; Dahan et al. 2019; Musfeldt et al. 2016). However, given the unpredictability of absorption and other pharmacokinetic changes associated with bariatric surgery and rapid weight loss, sub-therapeutic levels are also a theoretical possibility. Bingham et al. (2016) provided some guidance in managing lithium in bariatric patients based on their clinical experience. They suggest that: (1) weekly lithium level monitoring should start in the pre-operative liquid meal replacement phase; (2) all patients should have pre-operative lithium levels documented to establish their baseline; (3) in the immediate post-operative period, patients should be routinely monitored within the first post-operative week to identify potential complications early; (4) lithium levels should be measured weekly during the first 6 post-operative weeks, given the significant change to patients' oral intake and the potential for fluid shifts; (5) any bariatric surgery patients on lithium who are experiencing gastrointestinal symptoms (nausea, vomiting, diarrhea) should have a lithium level drawn as a precaution.

Treatment guidelines increasingly suggest that optimum management of bipolar disorder needs integration of pharmacotherapy with targeted psychotherapy. The main goals of adjunctive psychotherapy for bipolar disorder include the education of patients, and when possible, caregivers, strategies for the management of stress, the identification and intervention of early signs of recurrence, the enhancement of adherence with drug regimens, and how to keep regular lifestyle habits (e.g., regular sleep pattern and healthy nutrition). If these goals are important for all patients with bipolar disorder, they are even more important for those patients who undergo bariatric surgery and are requested to complete recommended follow-up after surgery.

KEY POINTS

The evidence thus far suggests that surgery is likely a safe option for patients with well-controlled bipolar disorder.

Unstable symptomatic bipolar disorder is an absolute contraindication for bariatric surgery.

For patients on lithium undergoing bariatric surgery, the perioperative period represents a high-risk time for clinically significant pharmacokinetic changes.

References

Ahmed AT, Warton EM, Schaefer CA, Shen L, McIntyre RS. The effect of bariatric surgery on psychiatric course among patients with bipolar disorder. Bipolar Disord. 2013;15(7):753–63. Epub 2013 Aug 5. PubMed PMID: 23909994; PubMed Central PMCID: PMC3844030. https://doi.org/10.1111/bdi.12109.

Alam A, Raouf S, Recio FO. Lithium toxicity following vertical sleeve gastrectomy: a case report. Clin Psychopharmacol Neurosci. 2016;14(3):318–20. PubMed PMID: 27489390; PubMed Central PMCID: PMC4977813. https://doi.org/10.9758/cpn.2016.14.3.318.

Amare AT, Schubert KO, Klingler-Hoffmann M, Cohen-Woods S, Baune BT. The genetic overlap between mood disorders and cardiometabolic diseases: a systematic review of genome wide and candidate gene studies. Transl Psychiatry. 2017;7(1):e1007. Review. PubMed PMID: 28117839; PubMed Central PMCID: PMC5545727. https://doi.org/10.1038/tp.2016.261.

Bingham KS, Thoma J, Hawa R, Sockalingam S. Perioperative lithium use in bariatric surgery: a case series and literature review. Psychosomatics. 2016;57(6):638–44. Epub 2016 Jul 15. Review. PubMed PMID: 27726858. https://doi.org/10.1016/j.psym.2016.07.001.

Boulanger H, Tebeka S, Girod C, Lloret-Linares C, Meheust J, Scott J, Guillaume S, Courtet P, Bellivier F, Delavest M. Binge eating behaviours in bipolar disorders. J Affect Disord. 2018;225:482–8. Epub 2017 Aug 31. PubMed PMID: 28865369. https://doi.org/10.1016/j. jad.2017.08.068.

Dahan A, Porat D, Azran C, Mualem Y, Sakran N, Abu-Abeid S. Lithium toxicity with severe bradycardia post sleeve gastrectomy: a case report and review of the literature. Obes Surg. 2019;29(2):735–8. PubMed PMID: 30448980. https://doi.org/10.1007/s11695-018-3597-x.

Fisher D, Coleman KJ, Arterburn DE, Fischer H, Yamamoto A, Young DR, Sherwood NE, Trinacty CM, Lewis KH. Mental illness in bariatric surgery: a cohort study from the PORTAL network. Obesity (Silver Spring). 2017;25(5):850–6. PubMed PMID: 28440047. https://doi. org/10.1002/oby.21814.

Friedman KE, Applegate K, Portenier D, McVay MA. Bariatric surgery in patients with bipolar spectrum disorders: selection factors, postoperative visit attendance, and weight outcomes. Surg Obes Relat Dis. 2017;13(4):643–51. Epub 2016 Oct 17. PubMed PMID: 28169206; PubMed Central PMCID: PMC5400728. https://doi.org/10.1016/j.soard.2016.10.009.

Grothe KB, Mundi MS, Himes SM, Sarr MG, Clark MM, Geske JR, Kalsy SA, Frye MA. Bipolar disorder symptoms in patients seeking bariatric surgery. Obes Surg. 2014;24(11):1909–14. PubMed PMID: 24752620. https://doi.org/10.1007/s11695-014-1262-6.

Kouidrat Y, Amad A, Stubbs B, Moore S, Gaughran F. Surgical management of obesity among people with schizophrenia and bipolar disorder: a systematic review of outcomes and recommendations for future research. Obes Surg. 2017;27(7):1889–95. Review. PubMed PMID: 28508277. https://doi.org/10.1007/s11695-017-2715-5.

Musfeldt D, Levinson A, Nykiel J, Carino G. Lithium toxicity after Roux-en-Y bariatric surgery. BMJ Case Rep. 2016;2016:bcr2015214056. PubMed PMID: 26994048; PubMed Central PMCID: PMC4800199. https://doi.org/10.1136/bcr-2015-214056.

Reilly-Harrington NA, Feig EH, Huffman JC. Bipolar disorder and obesity: contributing factors, impact on clinical course, and the role of bariatric surgery. Curr Obes Rep. 2018;7(4):294–300. Review. PubMed PMID: 30368736. https://doi.org/10.1007/s13679-018-0322-y.

Shelby SR, Labott S, Stout RA. Bariatric surgery: a viable treatment option for patients with severe mental illness. Surg Obes Relat Dis. 2015;11(6):1342–8. Epub 2015 Jun 3. PubMed PMID: 26363716. https://doi.org/10.1016/j.soard.2015.05.016.

Sicras A, Rejas J, Navarro R, Serrat J, Blanca M. Metabolic syndrome in bipolar disorder: a cross-sectional assessment of a Health Management Organization database. Bipolar Disord. 2008;10(5):607–16. PubMed PMID: 18657245. https://doi. org/10.1111/j.1399-5618.2008.00599.x.

Steinmann WC, Suttmoeller K, Chitima-Matsiga R, Nagam N, Suttmoeller NR, Halstenson NA. Bariatric surgery: 1-year weight loss outcomes in patients with bipolar and other psychiatric disorders. Obes Surg. 2011;21(9):1323–9. PubMed PMID: 21380795. https://doi. org/10.1007/s11695-011-0373-6.

Taylor VH, Misra M. Bariatric surgery in patients with bipolar disorder: an emerging issue. J Psychiatry Neurosci. 2009;34(4):E3–4. PubMed PMID: 19568475; PubMed Central PMCID: PMC2702441.

Psychotic Disorders

11

Abstract

Unlike eating and mood disorders, psychotic disorders have been scarcely investigated by studies focusing on the relationship between psychopathology and
bariatric surgery. That is unfortunate because the prevalence of severe obesity
and metabolic disorders is high among patients with psychotic syndromes and
bariatric surgery may be a viable treatment option for some of them. Although
psychosis is often mentioned as an absolute contraindication to bariatric surgery,
there is evidence that the outcomes of patients with schizophrenia spectrum disorders are comparable to those of patients with no pre-operative mental illness.
The diagnosis per se is not sufficient for deciding if bariatric surgery is a viable
treatment option for an individual patient with obesity and psychosis. The decision should be based on the assessment of many other dimensional variables that
impact surgery outcome more than categorical diagnosis. In addition to categorical diagnosis, pre-operative clinical assessment should focus on symptoms,
insight, reality testing, cognitive capacity, and functioning. Better surgery outcomes are more likely in patients with complete or significant remission of
symptoms, good insight, adequate reality testing, undamaged cognitive capacity,
and satisfactory functioning.

Keywords

Psychosis · Schizophrenia · Insight · Reality testing · Cognitive capacity

11.1 Background

Unlike eating and mood disorders, psychotic disorders have been scarcely investigated by studies focusing on the relationship between psychopathology and bariatric surgery. That is unfortunate because the prevalence of severe obesity and

© Springer Nature Switzerland AG 2020
A. Troisi, *Bariatric Psychology and Psychiatry*,
https://doi.org/10.1007/978-3-030-44834-9_11

metabolic disorders is high among patients with psychotic syndromes and bariatric surgery may be a viable treatment option for some of them.

A recent large-scale meta-analysis showed that almost 1 in 3 of unselected patients with schizophrenia suffers from metabolic syndrome and 1 in 2 are overweight (Mitchell et al. 2013). Patients with schizophrenia have higher intake of calories in the form of high-density food and lower energy expenditure. The etiology of obesity and metabolic disorders in this patient population is multifactorial, including psychosocial and socioeconomic risk factors, unhealthy lifestyle, pretreatment/premorbid genetic vulnerabilities, and adverse effects of antipsychotic drugs (Manu et al. 2015).

This chapter outlines basic notions on schizophrenia and other psychotic disorders; illustrates assessment procedures; and reviews published data on the indications, contraindications, and outcomes of bariatric surgery in patients with psychotic syndromes. The final section on clinical management synthetizes the information necessary to decide if to offer or not surgical treatment to this patient population.

11.2   Basic Notions

Schizophrenia is a severe mental disorder with a peak age of onset between 15 and 35 years. The incidence of schizophrenia is estimated to be 5 per 100,000 people. Males and females are equally affected, but men aged <45 years have twice the rate of schizophrenia as women. The main symptoms of schizophrenia are delusions, hallucinations, disorganized thinking, abnormal motor behavior, and negative symptoms. Delusions are fixed beliefs that are not amenable to change despite evidence to the contrary. Their content may include a variety of themes. An example of persecutory delusion is the belief that one is going to be harmed or harassed by a criminal or political organization. Hallucinations are perceptions in the absence of an external stimulus. They may occur in any sensory modality, but auditory hallucinations (e.g., hearing voices of running commentary nature) are the most common in schizophrenia. Disorganized thinking reflects abnormalities of the ways thoughts are linked together. During the interview, the patient may switch from one topic to another. Answers to questions may be marginally related or completely unrelated. Abnormal motor behavior may include a marked decrease in reactivity to the environment (catatonic behavior) or stereotyped movements (staring, grimacing, echoing of speech). Negative symptoms may include loss of drive for any social engagements (asociality), reduced ability to initiate goal-direct behavior (avolition), poverty of speech (alogia), and lack of pleasure in activities that were previously enjoyable to the patient (anhedonia).

In addition to schizophrenia, DSM-5 includes other psychotic disorders in the schizophrenia spectrum: delusional disorder, brief psychotic disorder, schizophreniform disorder, and schizoaffective disorder. In the field of bariatric surgery, the differences between one specific psychotic disorder and any other in the schizophrenia spectrum are scarcely relevant. What matters is the severity of reality distortion and the course of the disorder (i.e., acute with remission versus chronic with enduring

Table 11.1 Prognostic subtypes of psychotic disorders

CLINICAL FEATURE	GOOD PROGNOSIS	POOR PROGNOSIS
Family history	Negative	Positive
Onset	Acute	Gradual
IQ	Normal	Low
Premorbid functioning	Good	Poor
Stressors	Yes	No
Gender	Female	Male
Negative symptoms	Absent or mild	Prominent
Brain imaging	Normal	Abnormal

symptoms) (Table 11.1). Psychotic symptoms such as delusions and hallucinations can also be present in mood disorders (e.g., unipolar depression or bipolar disorder). Mood disorders and their relevance to bariatric surgery are discussed elsewhere in this book (see Chaps. 7 and 10). However, regardless of the DSM diagnosis, the presence of psychotic symptoms in candidates to bariatric surgery raises the same clinical problems. Thus, what said in this chapter about patients with schizophrenia spectrum disorders applies also to patients with mood disorders and psychotic symptoms.

Some psychotic syndromes fully remit spontaneously or after a variable period of treatment. However, most cases follow a chronic course and patients need long-term therapy with antipsychotic drugs. Antipsychotic drugs differ widely in terms of metabolic side effects. Choice of antipsychotic treatment is a critical aspect in patients seeking and undergoing bariatric surgery.

11.3 Assessment

There are many rating scales for assessing the presence and severity of psychotic symptoms, including the *Brief Psychiatric Rating Scale* (BPRS) and the *Positive and Negative Symptoms Scale* (PANSS). When administered by an experienced mental health clinician, these scales provide accurate and extensive information on the current mental status of bariatric candidates with a personal history of psychosis. The use of standardized rating scales is necessary to ascertain if the patient has achieved the level of symptomatic remission compatible with bariatric surgery. This is mandatory in patients with chronic psychotic disorders and enduring symptoms, even if they are stable and on pharmacologic treatment. In patients with a past history of acute psychotic disorder followed by complete and long-standing remission, it is useful to ask questions concerning residual symptoms: "Have you recently had the experience of hearing voices talking when there is nobody around?" "Are you afraid that someone else is trying to harm you?" "Have you recently felt that thoughts are being taken out of your mind?" "Have you recently felt under the control of an outside force?" Positive answers to one or more of these questions suggest the necessity of standardized assessment of mental status.

Insight is defined as a patient's capacity to understand the nature, significance, and severity of his or her illness. In clinical practice, patients with milder episodes of psychosis, who are aware of having a mental illness, will be reported to have good insight while those with severe illness, who solely believe in their delusional ideas, will be considered to lack such understanding. There are various scales for assessing the level of insight including the *Lack of Insight Index*, the *Insight Scale*, and the *Beck Cognitive Insight Scale*. Good insight is a prerequisite for adherence to follow-up programs and treatment prescriptions.

ASSESSMENT TIPS

Prognostic subtype is more important than DSM categorical diagnosis.

Assess current severity of psychotic symptoms.

Assess the capacity for reality testing.

Assess the level of insight.

11.4   Bariatric Data

Based on the meta-analysis published by Dawes et al. (2016), the prevalence rate of psychosis among patients seeking and undergoing bariatric surgery is very low (1%). This is an unexpected finding considering the high prevalence of severe obesity among patients with psychotic syndromes. Likely, the common opinion that psychosis is an absolute contraindication to bariatric surgery is a barrier even to pre-operative evaluation.

Archid et al. (2019) compared surgical and psychiatric outcomes of seven patients with schizophrenia and 59 mentally health patients 2 years after sleeve gastrectomy. The calculated excess weight loss (%EWL) showed no significant differences in both groups (51.68 ± 15.84% for patients with schizophrenia and 60.68 ± 19.95% for mentally health patients). The psychiatric status of the patients with schizophrenia was stable in all cases, and no exacerbation of psychiatric symptoms was observed during the time of follow-up.

Kouidrat et al. (2017) published a systematic review of the outcomes of bariatric surgery among patients with severe mental disorders (i.e., bipolar disorder or schizophrenia). The review was based on eight studies including a total of 279 participants. The mean length of follow-up was 15.7 months (range 12–24). Of the eight studies, two were prospective cohort studies and six involved a control group of participants without a psychiatric diagnosis. However, patients with a diagnosis of schizophrenia were a small minority ($N = 14$). Based on the studies reported in the review, the outcomes for the subgroup of bariatric patients with schizophrenia were positive. Hamoui et al. (2004) found no significant differences between schizophrenia patients and controls at 6 months. Excess weight loss (%EWL) was 39.5% (range 29.4–62.9%) in patients versus 46.9% (range 30.0–95.5%) in controls. Fuchs et al. (2016) found that the four schizophrenia patients had a 35.7% EWL, an outcome comparable to that of patients without any psychiatric comorbidity at 1 year. Finally, in the non-controlled study of Shelby et al. (2015), using 50% EWL as the standard for bariatric surgery success, all the three patients met this criterion.

Data related to post-surgery psychiatric status were mixed. In the study of Hamoui et al. (2004), no patient required psychiatric hospitalization following surgery and all continued to live at home with regular psychiatric follow-up. In the study of Shelby et al. (2015), the three schizophrenia patients experienced exacerbation of psychiatric problems such as agitation, paranoia, auditory hallucinations, and also medication changes. One required inpatient psychiatric hospitalization. Since patients with schizophrenia experience symptom fluctuations through the course of their illness, it is difficult to establish if psychotic exacerbation was a negative outcome of bariatric surgery.

To compare bariatric surgery (vertical sleeve gastrectomy or Roux-en-Y gastric bypass) outcomes according to preoperative mental illness category, Fisher et al. (2017) published a large retrospective cohort study including 8192 patients with a mean postoperative enrollment span of 2.9 years. The sample included 508 patients with a diagnosis of bipolar disorder, psychosis, or schizophrenia. Their weight loss was very similar to that recorded in patients with no preoperative mental illness. However, the subgroup of patients with severe mental illness had a greater acute care use (i.e., emergency department visits and hospital days) beginning as soon as 3 months after surgery and persisting through 2 years of follow-up. Several methodological problems make it difficult to translate these findings into clear clinical indications. First, the psychiatric diagnosis was derived from an algorithm combining clinical data with prescribed medications, not on a standardized interview. Second, the reasons for requiring post-operative acute care were not specified. Third, the study did not examine outcomes of other bariatric procedures such as adjustable gastric banding or duodenal switch. Fourth, and most important, patients with psychotic syndromes were combined with bipolar patients. Against these methodological limitations, the authors emphasized that their study population *represented a group that, despite mental illness history, had been cleared for surgery due to a clinical judgment that they were stable preoperatively.* (p. 856).

11.5 Clinical Management

In a large survey, 31% of mental health professionals reported psychotic disorders as a specific psychiatric contraindication to bariatric surgery (Fabricatore et al. 2006). According to an IFSO Consensus Statement, *surgery is a contraindication in cases of unstable schizophrenia and psychosis.* (De Luca et al. 2016). How can we reconcile these recommendations with the data reported in the previous section suggesting that the outcomes of patients with schizophrenia spectrum disorders are comparable to those of patients with no preoperative mental illness? The explanation is the clinical heterogeneity of psychotic syndromes. The diagnosis per se is not sufficient for deciding if bariatric surgery is a viable treatment option for an individual patient with obesity and psychosis. The decision should be based on the assessment of many other dimensional variables that impact surgery outcome more than categorical diagnosis. Two key variables are the severity of psychotic symptoms and the level of insight. Patients with hallucinations and/or delusions are unlikely to adhere to pre- and post-operative guidelines and have a high risk of worse outcomes (Sogg et al. 2016). Severe psychotic symptoms are associated with gross reality distortion that impairs patients' capacity to understand and follow prescribed clinical procedures. This is especially true for patients with scarce insight (i.e., awareness of illness).

In addition to categorical diagnosis, pre-operative clinical assessment should focus on symptoms, insight, reality testing, cognitive capacity, and functioning. Better surgery outcomes are more likely in patients with complete or significant remission of symptoms, good insight, adequate reality testing, undamaged cognitive capacity, and satisfactory functioning. In bariatric surgery, informed consent is a dynamic process based on a thorough discussion with the patient regarding the risks and the benefits, procedural options, choices of surgeon and medical institution, the need for nutritional and behavioral changes before and after surgery, and the need for long-term post-operative follow-up (Mechanick et al. 2013). If psychotic symptoms and scarce insight interfere with the patient's capacity to subscribe an informed consent including all the aspects listed above, bariatric surgery should be delayed or denied.

After surgery, patients with a history of psychosis should be assessed periodically to ensure an early diagnosis of psychotic relapse, optimize maintenance treatment (choice of antipsychotic drugs and measurement of blood levels), and evaluate adherence to nutritional and behavioral changes.

KEY POINTS

Bariatric surgery is a viable option for patients with a history of psychosis who have achieved stable remission.

Poor insight and compromised reality testing jeopardize the understanding of relevant information included in the informed consent.

Active psychosis is an absolute contraindication for bariatric surgery.

References

Archid R, Archid N, Meile T, Hoffmann J, Hilbert J, Wulff D, Teufel M, Muthig M, Quante M, Königsrainer A, Lange J. Patients with schizophrenia do not demonstrate worse outcome after sleeve gastrectomy: a short-term cohort study. Obes Surg. 2019;29(2):506–10. PubMed PMID: 30397877. https://doi.org/10.1007/s11695-018-3578-0.

Dawes AJ, Maggard-Gibbons M, Maher AR, Booth MJ, Miake-Lye I, Beroes JM, Shekelle PG. Mental health conditions among patients seeking and undergoing bariatric surgery: a meta-analysis. JAMA. 2016;315(2):150–63. PubMed PMID: 26757464. https://doi.org/10.1001/jama.2015.18118.

De Luca M, Angrisani L, Himpens J, Busetto L, Scopinaro N, Weiner R, Sartori A, Stier C, Lakdawala M, Bhasker AG, Buchwald H, Dixon J, Chiappetta S, Kolberg HC, Frühbeck G, Sarwer DB, Suter M, Soricelli E, Blüher M, Vilallonga R, Sharma A, Shikora S. Indications for surgery for obesity and weight-related diseases: position statements from the International Federation for the Surgery of Obesity and Metabolic Disorders (IFSO). Obes Surg. 2016;26(8):1659–96. PubMed PMID: 27412673; PubMed Central PMCID: PMC6037181. https://doi.org/10.1007/s11695-016-2271-4.

Fabricatore AN, Crerand CE, Wadden TA, Sarwer DB, Krasucki JL. How do mental health professionals evaluate candidates for bariatric surgery? Survey results. Obes Surg. 2006;16(5):567–73. PubMed PMID: 16687023.

Fisher D, Coleman KJ, Arterburn DE, Fischer H, Yamamoto A, Young DR, Sherwood NE, Trinacty CM, Lewis KH. Mental illness in bariatric surgery: a cohort study from the PORTAL network. Obesity (Silver Spring). 2017;25(5):850–6. PubMed PMID: 28440047. https://doi.org/10.1002/oby.21814.

Fuchs HF, Laughter V, Harnsberger CR, Broderick RC, Berducci M, DuCoin C, Langert J, Sandler BJ, Jacobsen GR, Perry W, Horgan S. Patients with psychiatric comorbidity can safely undergo bariatric surgery with equivalent success. Surg Endosc. 2016;30(1):251–8. Epub 2015 Apr 7. PubMed PMID: 25847138. https://doi.org/10.1007/s00464-015-4196-8.

Hamoui N, Kingsbury S, Anthone GJ, Crookes PF. Surgical treatment of morbid obesity in schizophrenic patients. Obes Surg. 2004;14(3):349–52. PubMed PMID: 15072656.

Kouidrat Y, Amad A, Stubbs B, Moore S, Gaughran F. Surgical management of obesity among people with schizophrenia and bipolar disorder: a systematic review of outcomes and recommendations for future research. Obes Surg. 2017;27(7):1889–95. Review. PubMed PMID: 28508277. https://doi.org/10.1007/s11695-017-2715-5.

Manu P, Dima L, Shulman M, Vancampfort D, De Hert M, Correll CU. Weight gain and obesity in schizophrenia: epidemiology, pathobiology, and management. Acta Psychiatr Scand. 2015;132(2):97–108. Epub 2015 May 27. Review. PubMed PMID: 26016380. https://doi.org/10.1111/acps.12445.

Mechanick JI, Youdim A, Jones DB, Garvey WT, Hurley DL, MM MM, Heinberg LJ, Kushner R, Adams TD, Shikora S, Dixon JB, Brethauer S, American Association of Clinical Endocrinologists; Obesity Society; American Society for Metabolic & Bariatric Surgery. Clinical practice guidelines for the perioperative nutritional, metabolic, and nonsurgical support of the bariatric surgery patient—2013 update: cosponsored by American Association of Clinical Endocrinologists, The Obesity Society, and American Society for Metabolic & Bariatric Surgery. Obesity (Silver Spring). 2013;21(Suppl 1):S1–27. PubMed PMID: 23529939; PubMed Central PMCID: PMC4142593. https://doi.org/10.1002/oby.20461.

Mitchell AJ, Vancampfort D, Sweers K, van Winkel R, Yu W, De Hert M. Prevalence of metabolic syndrome and metabolic abnormalities in schizophrenia and related disorders—a systematic review and meta-analysis. Schizophr Bull. 2013;39(2):306–18. Epub 2011 Dec 29. Review. PubMed PMID: 22207632; PubMed Central PMCID: PMC3576174. https://doi.org/10.1093/schbul/sbr148.

Shelby SR, Labott S, Stout RA. Bariatric surgery: a viable treatment option for patients with severe mental illness. Surg Obes Relat Dis. 2015;11(6):1342–8. Epub 2015 Jun 3. PubMed PMID: 26363716. https://doi.org/10.1016/j.soard.2015.05.016.

Sogg S, Lauretti J, West-Smith L. Recommendations for the presurgical psychosocial evaluation of bariatric surgery patients. Surg Obes Relat Dis. 2016;12(4):731–49. Epub 2016 Feb 12. Review. PubMed PMID: 27179400. https://doi.org/10.1016/j.soard.2016.02.008.

Intellectual Disability

12

Abstract

Until recently, a diagnosis of intellectual disability was an absolute contraindication to bariatric surgery. Such a conservative approach reflects a series of worries concerning the capacity of patients to understand the risks and benefits related to surgical procedures and their capacity and willingness to adhere to post-operative treatment guidelines. However, a recent review concluded that patients with intellectual disability who underwent bariatric surgery showed significant weight reduction immediately after bariatric surgery as well as improvements in behavioral problems, and cooperation. Some of these benefits were counterbalanced by major weight regain at long-term follow-up. Adequate and flexible pre-operative care incorporating a strong multidisciplinary team and regular consultation may contribute to achieve informed consent and strengthen patient–clinician collaboration. Pre-operative care should extend beyond the patient and incorporate their support networks. This may include providing specific psychiatric counseling to the families or caregivers as a means to foster unambiguous communication and reduce uncertainty throughout the process. Post-operative care should be modified to address the challenge of dietary compliance in this population. Waiting for the critical data that we currently lack, the decision to offer bariatric surgery to a patient with intellectual disability remains difficult and depends on an accurate evaluation of risks and benefits in each individual case.

Keywords

Intellectual disability · Contraindication · Informed consent · Dietary compliance Support network

12.1 Background

The prevalence of being overweight and obese among adults with intellectual disability is reportedly 28%–71% and 17%–43%, respectively. Factors increasing the susceptibility of being overweight or obese have been identified as female gender, increasing age, having a certain diagnosis (e.g., Down syndrome), mild intellectual disability, as well as living independently/with family (versus living in staffed residences), consuming certain prescription medications, and non-participation in physical activities (Ranjan et al. 2018). In the short term, combined interventions targeting different lifestyle risk factors have proved to be useful to decrease the prevalence and severity of obesity among persons with intellectual disability. However, weight reduction strategies are often unsuccessful when their efficacy is assessed over an extended period of time (Spanos et al. 2013). Thus, the possibility of offering surgical treatment for obesity to this group of patients is increasingly being viewed as one of the therapeutic alternatives to be taken into consideration.

This chapter outlines basic notions on intellectual disabilities; reviews published data on the indications, contraindications, and outcomes of bariatric surgery in patients with intellectual disabilities; and illustrates assessment procedures that can inform the clinical decision to offer or not surgical treatment to this patient population.

12.2 Basic Notions

DSM-5 defines intellectual disabilities as neurodevelopmental disorders that begin in childhood and are characterized by intellectual difficulties as well as difficulties in conceptual, social, and practical areas of living. The DSM-5 diagnosis of intellectual disabilities requires the satisfaction of three criteria: (1) deficits in intellectual functioning (i.e., reasoning, problem solving, planning, abstract thinking, judgment, academic learning, and learning from experience) confirmed by clinical evaluation and individualized standard IQ testing; (2) deficits in adaptive functioning that significantly hamper conforming to developmental and sociocultural standards for the individual's independence and ability to meet their social responsibility; and (3) the onset of these deficits during childhood.

DSM-5 emphasizes that the level of severity of intellectual disability should be defined on the basis of adaptive functioning, and not IQ scores. In practice, IQ scores are still largely used by clinicians to distinguish different levels of severity (IQ 50–70, mild; 35–49, moderate; 20–34, severe; <20, profound). Mild intellectual disability is not usually associated with specific causes and represents the lower end of the IQ normal distribution curve. More severe intellectual disability is generally related to brain damage and can be caused by a variety of pathogenic factors (genetic, infective, toxic, nutritional, metabolic) acting in the antenatal, perinatal, and postnatal developmental periods. Depending on the severity of the individual case, diagnostic assessment includes both standard intelligence tests (e.g., the *Wechsler Intelligence Scale for Children*, the *Wechsler Adult Intelligence Scale*, the

Table 12.1 Variables influencing eligibility to bariatric surgery in patients with intellectual disabilities

- IQ score
- Adaptive functioning
- Behavioral disturbance
- Psychiatric comorbidity
- Living environment
- Social support
- Professional support

Stanford-Binet Intelligence Scale) and measures of adaptive functioning (e.g., the *Vineland Adaptive Behavior Scales* or the *Adaptive Behavior Assessment System*).

Various medical and psychiatric comorbidities are often associated with intellectual disability (Kishore et al. 2019). Common medical comorbidities are the following: epilepsy, spasticity, dystonia, ataxia, visual impairment, hearing impairment, congenital heart disease, cleft lip and cleft palate, limb anomalies, congenital dislocation of hip joint, renal malformations, failure to thrive with vitamin and mineral deficiencies, recurrent infections, feeding disorder, and short stature. People with intellectual disability are 3–5 times at higher risk of any psychiatric disorder compared to the general population at all ages, with a cumulative prevalence of around 40%. The etiology of intellectual disability can often provide clues to anticipate certain psychiatric comorbidities as certain behavioral phenotypes are frequently associated with some syndromes. Some examples are severe self-injurious behavior in Lesch-Nyhan syndrome; skin picking and obsessive-compulsive disorder in Prader-Willi syndrome; autistic traits and hyperactivity in Fragile X syndrome; self-hugging stereotypy and trichotillomania in Smith-Magenis syndrome; schizophrenia-like disorders in 22q11 deletion syndrome. In most patients, unspecified behavioral disorders are very common. Obviously, the assessment for eligibility to bariatric surgery should take into consideration the presence of medical and psychiatric comorbidities (Table 12.1).

12.3 Bariatric Data

There are very few papers reporting on bariatric surgery in patients with intellectual disability. The scoping review by Gibbons et al. (2017) is currently the most informative source of clinical data in this area of bariatric surgery. The review analyzed 16 studies including a total of 49 patients. Eight studies (50%) were case series while the remaining six studies (50%) were case reports. No randomized control trials were reported in the literature. Four studies included an IQ score as a description of the patient sample ranging from 49 to 95. In all patients except one, the diagnosis associated with intellectual disability was Prader-Willi syndrome. Post-operative outcomes were measured using varied follow-up periods. Six (37.5%) interventions had post-operative follow-up periods of less than two years while the remaining studies had follow-ups ranging from 2 to 10 years. All 16 studies employed the degree of weight loss as the primary outcome measure. Weight loss in kilograms ranged from 1 to 63 kg. Weight loss outcomes were also measured in terms of percent of excess weight loss (%EWL). Results showed that %EWL ranged from 12% to 86%. Roux-en-Y gastric bypass and laparoscopic mini-gastric bypass produced the largest reported relative weight loss in terms of %EWL. Three studies described major weight regain by long-term follow-up including participants who underwent the biliopancreatic diversion procedure. Gibbons et al. (2017) concluded that patients with intellectual disability showed significant weight reduction immediately after bariatric surgery as well as improvements in behavioral problems and cooperation. However, some of these benefits were counterbalanced by major weight regain at long-term follow-up. Possible reasons for the less stable weight loss may include patients' resistance to dietary therapy and compulsive hyperphagia.

It is not clear if these conclusions apply only to patients with Prader-Willi syndrome or can be generalized to other intellectual disabilities. The results of some studies seem to support the former hypothesis. Liu et al. (2020) conducted a 10-year prospective observational study on five Prader-Willi patients who received bariatric surgery. The best mean percentage of total weight loss (%TWL) was achieved at 2 years (24.7%). %TWL dropped to 23.3% at 3 years, 11.9% at 5 years, 4.1% at 8 years, and 0% at 10 years. Each patient had at least three comorbidities preoperatively, but none of them had resolution of any one of the comorbidities at the last follow-up. The authors concluded that bariatric surgery could not produce sustainable long-term weight loss or comorbidity resolution in Prader-Willi syndrome.

In contrast with Liu et al.'s negative findings, Daigle et al. (2015) reported successful outcomes in six patients with intellectual disabilities other than Prader-Willi syndrome. The cohort (3 males, 3 females) had a mean age of 33.3 years and a mean BMI of 49.4. Two of the patients had a diagnosis of trisomy 21, and the other four patients had lifelong cognitive impairment from unknown causes. The distribution of surgical approaches was 2 laparoscopic Roux-en-Y gastric bypasses (RYGBs), 3 laparoscopic sleeve gastrectomies, and 1 laparoscopic adjustable gastric band (LAGB). There were no complications and no mortality. At a mean follow-up of 33.7 months, the cohort had a mean percent excess weight loss (%EWL) of 31.1% (range: 1.8%–72.2%). Two patients achieved a %EWL > 50%. In a prospective study of 64 adolescents who had received bariatric surgery, Hornack et al. (2019) found that having cognitive impairment or developmental disability did not significantly impact weight loss or weight loss trajectory in the 2 years after surgery. In addition, intelligence scores did not predict weight loss after surgery. The authors argued that having cognitive impairment or developmental disability should not be used as a criterion to deny surgery.

12.4 Clinical Management

Until recently, a diagnosis of intellectual disability was an absolute contraindication to bariatric surgery. In their recent review, Gibbons et al. (2017) reported that four out of five bariatric programs specify that severe intellectual disability is a definite contraindication while nearly half of these programs also consider a mild-to-moderate disability a definite contraindication. In the survey by Bauchowitz et al. (2005), only 6% of bariatric programs specify that mild–moderate levels of intellectual disability should not be considered a contraindication to surgical intervention. Such a conservative approach reflects a series of worries concerning the capacity of patients to understand the risks and benefits related to surgical procedures and their capacity and willingness to adhere to post-operative treatment guidelines. In addition, there is evidence that, among bariatric patients without intellectual disability, better baseline cognitive function is associated with better surgery outcomes (Spitznagel et al. 2013).

Future clinical research is expected to provide critical data that are currently missing and that are necessary to decide if bariatric surgery is a viable treatment option for the individual patient with intellectual disability. We need to know if the specific condition causing intellectual disability is more important than the IQ score. Findings from studies of patients with Prader-Willi syndrome seem to confirm that this may be the case. The hyperphagia and food obsession associated with such a syndrome do not remit after surgery and are likely to cause poor outcomes. Severe problems with eating behavior are not necessarily present in the behavioral profiles of other forms of intellectual disability, and such a difference may lead to better outcomes. We need to know if intensive and multidisciplinary intervention programs before and after surgery can compensate the limited capacity for self-management of patients with intellectual disability. Adequate and flexible pre-operative care incorporating a strong multidisciplinary team and regular consultation may contribute to achieve informed consent and strengthen patient–clinician collaboration. Pre-operative care should extend beyond the patient and incorporate their support networks. This may include providing specific psychiatric counseling to the families or caregivers as a means to foster unambiguous communication and reduce uncertainty throughout the process. Post-operative care should be modified to address the challenge of dietary compliance in this population. One strategy advocated by Heinberg and Schauer (2014) involved adjusting the frequency of follow-up with nutritionists and psychologists through the incorporation of monthly rather than quarterly visits. Finally, we need to know if bariatric surgery can improve cognitive functioning in patients with intellectual disability as is the case in patients without intellectual disability (Handley et al. 2016).

Waiting for the critical data that we currently lack, the decision to offer bariatric surgery to a patient with intellectual disability remains difficult and depends on an accurate evaluation of risks and benefits in each individual case.

KEY POINTS

Many bariatric programs indicate intellectual disability as a definite or possible contraindication to bariatric surgery.

Psychiatric comorbidity and behavioral disturbance are probably more important than IQ score in assessing eligibility to bariatric surgery.

Patients undergoing surgery require intensive pre- and post-operative treatment interventions including counseling to families and caregivers.

References

Bauchowitz AU, Gonder-Frederick LA, Olbrisch ME, Azarbad L, Ryee MY, Woodson M, Miller A, Schirmer B. Psychosocial evaluation of bariatric surgery candidates: a survey of present practices. Psychosom Med. 2005;67(5):825–32. PubMed PMID: 16204445.

Daigle CR, Schauer PR, Heinberg LJ. Bariatric surgery in the cognitively impaired. Surg Obes Relat Dis. 2015;11(3):711–4. Epub 2015 Feb 20. Review. PubMed PMID: 26093770. https://doi.org/10.1016/j.soard.2015.02.014.

Gibbons E, Casey AF, Brewster KZ. Bariatric surgery and intellectual disability: furthering evidence-based practice. Disabil Health J. 2017;10(1):3–10. Epub 2016 Sep 16. Review. PubMed PMID: 27720223. https://doi.org/10.1016/j.dhjo.2016.09.005.

Handley JD, Williams DM, Caplin S, Stephens JW, Barry J. Changes in cognitive function following bariatric surgery: a systematic review. Obes Surg. 2016;26(10):2530–7. Review. PubMed PMID: 27468905. https://doi.org/10.1007/s11695-016-2312-z.

Heinberg LJ, Schauer PR. Intellectual disability and bariatric surgery: a case study on optimization and outcome. Surg Obes Relat Dis. 2014;10(6):e105–8. Epub 2014 Jan 28. PubMed PMID: 24954542. https://doi.org/10.1016/j.soard.2014.01.014.

Hornack SE, Nadler EP, Wang J, Hansen A, Mackey ER. Sleeve gastrectomy for youth with cognitive impairment or developmental disability. Pediatrics. 2019;143(5):e20182908. Epub 2019 Apr 15. PubMed PMID: 30988024. https://doi.org/10.1542/peds.2018-2908.

Kishore MT, Udipi GA, Seshadri SP. Clinical practice guidelines for assessment and management of intellectual disability. Indian J Psychiatry. 2019;61(Suppl 2):194–210. PubMed PMID: 30745696; PubMed Central PMCID: PMC6345136. https://doi.org/10.4103/psychiatry.IndianJPsychiatry_507_18.

Liu SY, Wong SK, Lam CC, Ng EK. Bariatric surgery for Prader-Willi syndrome was ineffective in producing sustainable weight loss: long term results for up to 10 years. Pediatr Obes. 2020;15(1):e12575. Epub 2019 Sep 12. PubMed PMID: 31515962. https://doi.org/10.1111/ijpo.12575.

Ranjan S, Nasser JA, Fisher K. Prevalence and potential factors associated with overweight and obesity status in adults with intellectual developmental disorders. J Appl Res Intellect Disabil. 2018;31(Suppl 1):29–38. Epub 2017 May 24. Review. PubMed PMID: 28544175. https://doi.org/10.1111/jar.12370.

Spanos D, Melville CA, Hankey CR. Weight management interventions in adults with intellectual disabilities and obesity: a systematic review of the evidence. Nutr J. 2013;12:132. Review. PubMed PMID: 24060348; PubMed Central PMCID: PMC3849062. https://doi.org/10.1186/1475-2891-12-132.

Spitznagel MB, Garcia S, Miller LA, Strain G, Devlin M, Wing R, Cohen R, Paul R, Crosby R, Mitchell JE, Gunstad J. Cognitive function predicts weight loss after bariatric surgery. Surg Obes Relat Dis. 2013;9(3):453–9. Epub 2011 Oct 29. PubMed PMID: 22133580; PubMed Central PMCID: PMC3294182. https://doi.org/10.1016/j.soard.2011.10.008.

Substance and Alcohol Use Disorders

13

Abstract

There is much evidence that bariatric surgery can worsen the course of a preexistent substance use disorder or even cause its new onset post-operatively. Factors associated with new onset or increased substance use include the type of surgery, a personal history of substance use disorder, a family history of substance use disorder, a history of early trauma, pre-existing psychiatric disorders, low social support, younger age, male sex, and alcohol sensitization after surgery. Active substance abuse is considered a reason to exclude a patient from surgery by many guidelines. However, the decision to pursue surgery involves weighing the risks and benefits in each single case. A prudent clinical approach requires that the pre-surgical screening program identifies persons affected by such problems and allows them to receive treatment so that they can overcome the addiction and then be considered for weight loss surgery in the future.

Keywords

Substance use disorder · Alcohol · Illicit drugs · Altered pharmacokinetics · Brain reward systems · Addiction transfer

13.1 Background

There is much evidence that bariatric surgery can worsen the course of a preexistent substance use disorder or even cause its new onset post-operatively. The mechanisms linking bariatric surgery and substance use disorders are not fully understood, and more research is needed to identify the multiple pathogenic pathways that mediate post-surgery increased risk. In clinical practice, it is mandatory to investigate current and lifetime presence of substance use disorders in all patients seeking

© Springer Nature Switzerland AG 2020
A. Troisi, *Bariatric Psychology and Psychiatry*,
https://doi.org/10.1007/978-3-030-44834-9_13

surgical treatment for obesity and to monitor drug and alcohol use post-operatively, especially after the first 2 years post-surgery.

This chapter outlines basic notions on the classification, diagnosis, and treatment of substance use disorders; reviews data on their prevalence in bariatric patients before and after surgery; analyzes possible mechanisms linking bariatric surgery and substance use disorders; and summarizes the basic principles of clinical management to be implemented pre- and post-operatively.

13.2   Basic Notions

According to DSM-5, the essential feature of substance use disorders is a cluster of cognitive, behavioral, and physiological symptoms indicating that the patient continues using the substance despite significant substance-related problems. The pathological pattern of behaviors related to the use of the substance reflects impaired control and is associated with social impairment and risky use. An example of impaired control is when the patient takes the substance in larger amounts or over a longer period than was originally intended. Social impairment is evident when recurrent substance use results in a failure to fulfill major role obligations at work, school, or home. Risky use may consist of physical or mental problems caused by the substance that, despite their harmful consequences, do not bring the patient to abstain from using the substance (e.g., driving while intoxicated). According to DSM-5, the substances that can be used by patients with a diagnosis of substance use disorders belong to ten different classes. The likelihood that the patient will show the pharmacological phenomena of tolerance (i.e., necessity to increase doses to obtain the desired effect) and withdrawal (physical and mental symptoms caused by declining blood concentrations after prolonged heavy use) varies with the type of substance used (e.g., withdrawal symptoms are common with alcohol and opioids and absent with hallucinogens).

In common clinical language, "addiction" is often used as synonymous for substance use disorder, and "drugs" is the collective term used to indicate the psychoactive substances misused by patients with substance use disorders. Prevalence rates worldwide vary widely and are related to overall consumption levels (especially for alcohol), availability, and price. Among drugs, cannabis is the most common illicit substance used, followed by cocaine, and other stimulants.

The diagnosis of substance use disorder is based primarily on an assessment interview that aims at obtaining a clear history of drug use from the patient. Obviously, honest information from the patient is essential to collect valid data. The interview is organized around several questions: (1) Which substance(s)? (2) Which quantity? (3) How often? (4) For how long? (5) By what route (oral, smoke, etc.)? (6) Age when first started? (7) Which harmful consequences? (8) Previous treatments? When drug use is suspected but denied by the patient, drug screen tests can be requested. Compared to urine drug screen, saliva drug tests have a much shorter detection period, particularly for cannabis use. When diagnosing a substance use disorder, the clinician should investigate the possibility that the disorder is secondary to another mental disorder which requires specific treatment (e.g., alcohol abuse in bipolar disorder).

Interview can be combined with questionnaires. The *Alcohol Use Disorders Identification Test* (AUDIT) is a 10-item screening tool developed by the World Health Organization to assess alcohol consumption, drinking behaviors, and alcohol-related problems. Both a clinician-administered version and a self-report version of the AUDIT are available. A score of 8 or more indicates hazardous or harmful alcohol use. The CAGE is a very brief questionnaire based on four questions related to alcohol misuse: Have you ever felt you needed to cut down on your drinking? Have people annoyed you by criticizing your drinking? Have you ever felt guilty about drinking? Have you ever felt you needed a drink first thing in the morning (eye-opener) to steady your nerves or to get rid of a hangover? Two "yes" responses indicate that the possibility of alcoholism should be investigated further. The *Drug Use Questionnaire* (DAST-10) includes ten yes/no questions investigating potential involvement with drugs excluding alcohol and tobacco during the past 12 months. People with drug use problems score 3 or higher.

The essential components of addiction treatment are: harm minimization, motivational interviewing, solution-focused therapy, and relapse prevention, which is a form of cognitive behavioral therapy (CBT). Detoxification is required only where physiological tolerance to a drug has occurred. It enables patients to stop using the drug without experiencing withdrawal symptoms. Rehabilitation, either residential or involving daily attendance, can be useful in the later stages of the recovery process. Patients should be abstinent from drugs and show clear motivation to change their lifestyle before entering a rehabilitation program. It is important that, before approaching abstinence, patients are fully prepared for life without drugs.

Assessment tips
When diagnosing substance use disorder, specify which is/are the misused substance(s).
Assess both personal and family history of substance use disorder.
Ascertain if substance use disorder is secondary to, or comorbid with, another psychiatric disorder.
If drug use is suspected but denied by the patient, drug screen tests can be requested.

13.3   Bariatric Data

The lifetime prevalence of substance abuse disorders may be higher among obese patients seeking bariatric surgery compared with obese patients in the community (32.6% vs. 14.6%). However, very few patients (1.7%) meet diagnostic criteria for substance abuse disorder, including alcohol use disorder, at the time of the initial psychosocial evaluation (Parikh et al. 2016). These prevalence data point to the complexity of collecting reliable diagnostic information in bariatric candidates who are worried about not getting surgery.

13.3.1 Post-surgery Substance Use

As for the studies published between 1990 and 2015, the review by Li and Wu (2016) is the most comprehensive source of data on substance use after bariatric surgery. Forty studies were included in the review. Pre-operative history of substance use was a reliable predictor of post-operative substance use. The prevalence of post-operative alcohol use was higher among patients with pre-operative history of alcohol use than those without. Post-operative prevalence of alcohol use ranged from 7.6 to 11.8%. The proportion of new-onset substance users after surgery ranged from 34.3 to 89.5%. Among adults with no prior use history, certain types of drugs (opiate, benzodiazepine) were more likely to be initiated after surgery compared to alcohol and cigarettes. Relapsed users tended to use more types of substances (including initiating the use of a different substance) than new-onset users.

Other important studies have been published after the publication of the review by Li and Wu (2016). King et al. (2017) analyzed the data of the Longitudinal Assessment of Bariatric Surgery-2 (LABS-2) study, which is a prospective observational cohort study of patients at least 18 years old undergoing a first bariatric surgical procedure at ten hospitals from six clinical centers throughout the United States. The aim of the study was to evaluate alcohol consumption, symptoms of alcohol use disorder as measured by the AUDIT, illicit drug use (cocaine, hallucinogens, inhalants, phencyclidine, amphetamines, or marijuana), and treatment (counseling or hospitalization for alcohol or drugs) of substance use disorders before surgery and annually for 7 years following Roux-en-Y gastric bypass (RYGB) or laparoscopic adjustable gastric band (LAGB). The prevalence of alcohol use disorder increased substantially over time following RYGB from approximately 7% pre-surgery to 16% after 7 years, while remaining stable following LAGB between 6% and 8%. RYGB was associated with approximately twice the risk of incident alcohol use disorder and illicit drug use and nearly quadruple the risk of incident substance use disorder treatment over 7 years of follow-up. Male sex and younger age were identified as risk factors for incident alcohol use disorder and illicit drug use, while low income was associated with incident illicit drug use only. Different psychiatric variables were predictive of incident alcohol use disorder (i.e., less social support) and illicit drug use (i.e., anti-depressant medication use, history of psychiatric hospitalization). Contrary to the "addiction transfer" hypothesis (see below), pre-surgery binge eating and loss of control eating were not associated with an increased risk of post-surgery substance use disorder.

Kanji et al. (2019) conducted a systematic review to investigate the impact of bariatric surgery on weight loss outcomes, post-surgery substance use patterns, and other morbidity/mortality in patients with a history of substance use or substance use disorder. Fifty-eight studies were included in the review. Studies reporting weight loss after bariatric surgery did not demonstrate an association between substance use and negative weight loss outcomes. Several studies reported a significant portion of participants having new onset or increased substance use after bariatric surgery. Factors associated with new onset or increased substance use or substance use disorder included the type of surgery, a history of substance use disorder, a family history of substance use disorder, coping skills/life stressors, age, male sex, and alcohol sensitization after surgery. The authors of the review concluded that while substance use history does not appear to influence post-surgery weight loss, it may contribute to increased substance use after bariatric surgery.

Ibrahim et al. (2019) have recently published a prospective study comparing the effect of two different types of bariatric surgery (RYGB vs. sleeve grastrectomy) on alcohol use disorder. In their large sample ($N = 5724$), the percentage of patients with alcohol use disorder following RYGB increased from 7.6% at baseline to 11.9% at 2 years post-operatively, while the percentage of patients with alcohol use disorder following sleeve grastrectomy increased from 10.1% at baseline to 14.4% at 2 years post-operatively. Both procedures revealed a decrease in the percentage of patients with alcohol use disorder between baseline and 1 year post-operatively. Yet, in the second year after surgery, there were statistically significant increases in the development of new-onset alcohol use disorder for both sleeve gastrectomy (8.5%) and RYGB (7.2%). Predisposing factors to alcohol use disorder development for patients undergoing RYGB included higher household income, lower educational level, and any baseline alcohol consumption. For sleeve gastrectomy patients, any baseline alcohol consumption was associated with higher alcohol use disorder risk, while a pre-operative diagnosis of depression was associated with lower alcohol use disorder risk.

Although the majority of studies on post-surgery substance misuse have focused on alcohol (e.g., Smith et al. 2018), there is evidence that the problem can involve other drugs of abuse. Wallén et al. (2018) conducted a retrospective cohort study, including all patients undergoing gastric bypass surgery in Sweden between May 2007 and November 2013, to analyze the pattern of opioid use over time following gastric bypass surgery. They found an increase in the consumption of opioid analgesics. There was no difference in the use of opioid analgesics between women and men. The increase in the number of individuals with high opioid consumption in the total population was mainly due to an increase in the group of patients with a low consumption prior to surgery. Mean daily opioid consumption remained unchanged in the group with high consumption prior to surgery.

13.3.2 Mechanisms

The mechanisms linking bariatric surgery and substance use disorders are not fully understood. Several hypotheses have been advanced to explain post-surgery increased risk. Prevalent explanations focus on altered pharmacokinetics induced by the anatomical and physiological changes that result from surgical procedures. After RYGB and sleeve gastrectomy, there is a reduction in available gastric surface area. As a consequence, there is a decreased functionality of the metabolic enzyme gastric alcohol dehydrogenase, which is normally responsible for a small but significant amount of pre-systemic alcohol metabolism. The gastric emptying rate associated with liquids is also generally accelerated by RYGB and sleeve gastrectomy. This allows alcohol to reach the jejunum rapidly after ingestion where it is readily absorbed. There are also obvious changes in body weight that result from surgery, which alter the gram-per-kilogram dose of a fixed amount of alcohol given before and after surgery. In accord with such a hypothesis, research has shown that RYGB patients rapidly achieve peak blood alcohol concentrations that are significantly higher than expected in matched nonsurgical or pre-surgical comparison groups (Steffen et al. 2015).

However, heightened subjective sensitivity to alcohol due to altered pharmacokinetics is not the only possible explanation for substance use disorder after bariatric surgery. Studies with animal models support the hypothesis that RYGB increases the rewarding effects of alcohol independent of its direct gastric effects or change in alcohol absorption after the surgery. RYGB-treated obese rats increase intravenous alcohol administration, thus, through a route of administration where the stomach is bypassed.

Emphasis on altered pharmacokinetics does not explain post-surgery misuse of drugs taken via parenteral routes (transdermal, inhalation, intravenous) and neglects the importance of gut-brain communication. Brutman et al. (2019) reviewed recent findings showing that physical restructuring of the gastro-intestinal tract during bariatric surgery alters the secretion of feeding peptides and nutrient-sensing mechanisms that directly target the mesolimbic dopamine system (i.e., the brain circuitry that mediates hedonic response). Post-surgical changes in gastro-intestinal physiology augment the activation of the mesolimbic system. In some patients, this process may contribute to a reduced appetite for palatable food whereas in others it may support maladaptive motivated behavior for food and chemical drugs (Blackburn et al. 2017). Brain imaging studies in RYGB patients have demonstrated a decrease in dopamine D2 receptor availability in the ventral striatum and caudate nucleus after surgery. Dopamine has been termed "the pleasure neurotransmitter." It is possible that post-surgery changes in the functionality of the brain reward pathways increase the risk of misusing those substances (not only alcohol) that trigger subjective hedonic responses.

13.3.3 Patients' Perspectives

How do patients explain the link between bariatric surgery and substance misuse? Ivezaj et al. (2012) interviewed 24 patients who had undergone RYGB surgery and were admitted to a voluntary substance abuse treatment program. The aim of the study was to record patients' impressions of how their post-surgical substance use disorders emerged. Based on the patients' perceptions, four themes emerged regarding the etiology of substance use disorders, namely, unresolved psychological problems (*After losing weight, I was still left with issues. It was a roller-coaster of emotions...I was a fat person in a skinny person's body.*), addiction transfer (*I gave up love for food, and compensated that with going out and drinking.*), faster onset or stronger effects from substances (*A slam of wine felt just like a shot of heroin.*), and increased availability of pain medications (*Pain pills seemed safe and innocent...I began to act the part of a patient who was in pain in order to get more pills.*). 75% of the sample acknowledged unresolved psychological problems, 83.33% identified addiction transfer/substitution, 58.33% identified faster onset or stronger effects from substances, and 45.83% identified increased availability of pain medications. This is an important study because it highlights the complexity of the link between bariatric surgery and substance misuse and prompts clinicians to investigate patients' perceptions of what happens after surgery.

13.3.4 Addiction Transfer

After many years of successful bariatric surgeries, clinicians are now reporting that some patients are replacing compulsive overeating with newly acquired compulsive disorders such as alcoholism, gambling, drugs, and other addictions like compulsive shopping and exercise (Yoder et al. 2018). This unwanted effect of bariatric surgery has been termed "addiction transfer" or "cross-addiction" (Bak et al. 2016). The concept of a substitute behavior that serves the same purpose as the one it replaced is core to the hypothesis of addiction transfer. The hypothesis assumes that, being physically prevented from comfort eating after bariatric surgery, some patients employ substances or compulsive behaviors as a way to manage the problem of their unmet emotional and psychological needs.

The hypothesis of addiction transfer may be useful to explain what happens after surgery to those patients with preexistent disordered eating and/or depression, anxiety, post-traumatic stress disorder, and low self-esteem. However, it is applicability to the general population of bariatric patients with post-surgery substance misuse is questionable. The neurobiological mechanisms activated by gut-brain communication and described in the Sect. 13.3.2 may trigger substance misuse also in patients who did not employ comfort eating to counteract unpleasant emotions pre-operatively. In addition, long-term studies of substance misuse after bariatric surgery indicate that these problems tend to develop after a relatively long latency following surgery, typically about 1–2 years after surgery, and some evidence suggests that the risk for onset of such problems continues to increase, rather than decrease, over many years following surgery. If patients were experiencing a need to replace food and eating with some other type of substance or behavior, we would expect this need to be most acute within the early months after surgery, when patients are most limited in their intake capacity and their tolerance for highly palatable foods (Ivezaj et al. 2019).

13.4   Clinical Management

Post-surgery substance use disorders are emerging as one of the most critical psychiatric complications of bariatric surgery. Considering that risk factors have been consistently described (Table 13.1), pre-operative assessment should aim to identify

Table 13.1 Risk factors for post-surgery substance use disorder

• Personal history of substance abuse
• Family history of substance abuse
• History of early trauma
• Younger age
• Male sex
• Low social support
• Antidepressant medication use
• Smoking
• RYGB and sleeve gastrectomy

at-risk individuals and develop appropriate after-care plans associated with their recovery and progress throughout the bariatric process. After-care plans should be preceded by detailed information given to patients before surgery. In the study of Ivezaj et al. (2012) analyzing patients' impressions, over two thirds of the sample recommended that there should be increased knowledge regarding the associated risks of substance abuse post-surgery. Patients reported that there was not enough education, if any, on the risks of substance use following bariatric surgery. Clinicians should be aware that patients considering bariatric surgery in general and gastric bypass in particular should be informed of the possible risks regarding post-operative substance abuse.

Bariatric surgery patients may be at an elevated risk of needing pain medications due to postsurgical complications necessitating further surgery (e.g., hernia repairs, strictures, gall bladder, nicked nerves, and cosmetic surgery). Due to the altered neurobiological mechanisms of reward previously mentioned and increased need for pain medication following surgery, clinicians should be aware and cautious of distributing pain medications without proper education and follow-up care for their bariatric patients.

Active substance abuse is considered a reason to exclude a patient from surgery by many guidelines (e.g., Fried et al. 2013). Nonetheless, the decision to pursue surgery involves weighing the risks and benefits in each single case, and many patients with alcohol and/or drug abuse have undergone bariatric surgery, as indicated by the studies reviewed in the previous sections. A prudent clinical approach requires that the pre-surgical screening program identifies persons affected by such problems and allows them to receive treatment so that they can overcome the addiction and then be considered for weight loss surgery in the future.

KEY POINTS
Bariatric patients are particularly vulnerable to substance use disorders.
Pre-operative substance use is a reliable predictor of post-operative substance use.
Pre-operative and post-operative care should include interventions to prevent substance use disorders.
Patients considering bariatric surgery in general and gastric bypass in particular should be informed of the possible risks regarding post-operative substance use.

References

Bak M, Seibold-Simpson SM, Darling R. The potential for cross-addiction in post-bariatric surgery patients: Considerations for primary care nurse practitioners. J Am Assoc Nurse Pract. 2016;28(12):675–82. Epub 2016 Jul 11. PubMed PMID: 27400415. https://doi.org/10.1002/2327-6924.12390.

Blackburn AN, Hajnal A, Leggio L. The gut in the brain: the effects of bariatric surgery on alcohol consumption. Addict Biol. 2017;22(6):1540–53. Epub 2016 Aug 31. Review. PubMed PMID: 27578259; PubMed Central PMCID: PMC5332539. https://doi.org/10.1111/adb.12436.

Brutman JN, Sirohi S, Davis JF. Recent advances in the neurobiology of altered motivation following bariatric surgery. Curr Psychiatry Rep. 2019;21(11):117. Review. PubMed PMID: 31707546. https://doi.org/10.1007/s11920-019-1084-2.

Fried M, Yumuk V, Oppert JM, Scopinaro N, Torres AJ, Weiner R, Yashkov Y, Frühbeck G, European Association for the Study of Obesity; International Federation for the Surgery of Obesity—European Chapter. Interdisciplinary European Guidelines on metabolic and bariatric surgery. Obes Facts. 2013;6(5):449–68. Epub 2013 Oct 11. PubMed PMID: 24135948; PubMed Central PMCID: PMC5644681. https://doi.org/10.1159/000355480.

Ibrahim N, Alameddine M, Brennan J, Sessine M, Holliday C, Ghaferi AA. New onset alcohol use disorder following bariatric surgery. Surg Endosc. 2019;33(8):2521–30. Epub 2018 Oct 22. PubMed PMID: 30350107. https://doi.org/10.1007/s00464-018-6545-x.

Ivezaj V, Saules KK, Wiedemann AA. "I didn't see this coming.": why are postbariatric patients in substance abuse treatment? Patients' perceptions of etiology and future recommendations. Obes Surg. 2012;22(8):1308–14. PubMed PMID: 22661046. https://doi.org/10.1007/s11695-012-0668-2.

Ivezaj V, Benoit SC, Davis J, Engel S, Lloret-Linares C, Mitchell JE, Pepino MY, Rogers AM, Steffen K, Sogg S. Changes in alcohol use after metabolic and bariatric surgery: predictors and mechanisms. Curr Psychiatry Rep. 2019;21(9):85. Review. PubMed PMID: 31410716. https://doi.org/10.1007/s11920-019-1070-8.

Kanji S, Wong E, Akioyamen L, Melamed O, Taylor VH. Exploring pre-surgery and post-surgery substance use disorder and alcohol use disorder in bariatric surgery: a qualitative scoping review. Int J Obes (Lond). 2019;43(9):1659–74. Epub 2019 Jun 18. Erratum in: Int J Obes (Lond). 2019 Nov;43(11):2348. PubMed PMID: 31213657. https://doi.org/10.1038/s41366-019-0397-x.

King WC, Chen JY, Courcoulas AP, Dakin GF, Engel SG, Flum DR, Hinojosa MW, Kalarchian MA, Mattar SG, Mitchell JE, Pomp A, Pories WJ, Steffen KJ, White GE, Wolfe BM, Yanovski SZ. Alcohol and other substance use after bariatric surgery: prospective evidence from a U.S. multicenter cohort study. Surg Obes Relat Dis. 2017;13(8):1392–402. Epub 2017 Mar 31. PubMed PMID: 28528115; PubMed Central PMCID: PMC5568472. https://doi.org/10.1016/j.soard.2017.03.021.

Li L, Wu LT. Substance use after bariatric surgery: a review. J Psychiatr Res. 2016;76:16–29. Epub 2016 Jan 22. Review. PubMed PMID: 26871733; PubMed Central PMCID: PMC4789154. https://doi.org/10.1016/j.jpsychires.2016.01.009.

Parikh M, Johnson JM, Ballem N, American Society for Metabolic and Bariatric Surgery Clinical Issues Committee. ASMBS position statement on alcohol use before and after bariatric surgery. Surg Obes Relat Dis. 2016;12(2):225–30. Epub 2015 Nov 3. Review. PubMed PMID: 26968500. https://doi.org/10.1016/j.soard.2015.10.085.

Smith KE, Engel SG, Steffen KJ, Garcia L, Grothe K, Koball A, Mitchell JE. Problematic alcohol use and associated characteristics following bariatric surgery. Obes Surg. 2018;28(5):1248–54. PubMed PMID: 29110243; PubMed Central PMCID: PMC6483819. https://doi.org/10.1007/s11695-017-3008-8.

Steffen KJ, Engel SG, Wonderlich JA, Pollert GA, Sondag C. Alcohol and other addictive disorders following bariatric surgery: prevalence, risk factors and possible etiologies. Eur Eat Disord Rev. 2015;23(6):442–50. Epub 2015 Oct 8. Review. PubMed PMID: 26449524. https://doi.org/10.1002/erv.2399.

Wallén S, Szabo E, Palmetun-Ekbäck M, Näslund I. Use of opioid analgesics before and after gastric bypass surgery in Sweden: a population-based study. Obes Surg. 2018;28(11):3518–23. PubMed PMID: 29998381. https://doi.org/10.1007/s11695-018-3377-7.

Yoder R, MacNeela P, Conway R, Heary C. How do individuals develop alcohol use disorder after bariatric surgery? A grounded theory exploration. Obes Surg. 2018;28(3):717–24. PubMed PMID: 29032488. https://doi.org/10.1007/s11695-017-2936-7.

Suicide and Self-Harm

14

Abstract

There is a growing concern that post-bariatric surgery patients may have an increased risk for completed suicide, attempted suicide, and self-harm compared to age-, sex-, and BMI-matched controls. Although the pathogenic mechanisms increasing the risk are not fully understood, there is evidence that various pre- and post-surgical psychosocial, pharmacokinetic, physiologic, and medical factors may be involved. Mental health problems are much more prevalent in patients undergoing bariatric surgery than in age, gender, and BMI-matched controls. The high prevalence of preexisting psychiatric disorders combined with surgery-related changes may cause an increased risk of suicide and self-harm. Lifetime history of suicide ideation and self-injurious behavior are most strongly associated with post-surgery risk. Therefore, pre-operative assessment conducted by an expert mental health professional is crucial for effective prevention of self-harm and suicide in bariatric patients. Pre-operative assessment is very important, but it should be combined with post-operative assessment. Most programs focus on the first year post surgery, but there is evidence to support the call for long-term follow-up, especially for patients with a history of major depression, personality disorder, and/or self-injurious behavior.

Keywords

Suicide · Self-harm · Post-surgery risk · Pathogenic mechanisms · Long-term follow-up

© Springer Nature Switzerland AG 2020

A. Troisi, *Bariatric Psychology and Psychiatry*,

https://doi.org/10.1007/978-3-030-44834-9_14

14.1   Background

There is a growing concern that post-bariatric surgery patients may have an increased risk for completed suicide, attempted suicide, and self-harm compared to age-, sex-, and BMI-matched controls (Courcoulas 2017; Dixon 2016). Although the pathogenic mechanisms increasing the risk are not fully understood, there is evidence that various pre- and post-surgical psychosocial, pharmacokinetic, physiologic, and medical factors may be involved (Müller et al. 2019).

This chapter outlines basic notions on suicide and self-harm, reviews published data on increased risk in post-bariatric surgery patients, discusses the role of potential pathogenic mechanisms, and illustrates assessment methods and preventive strategies useful to reduce the risk of post-operative suicide and self-harm.

14.2   Basic Notions

14.2.1 Deliberate Self-Harm (DSH)

Self-harm has been defined as a preoccupation with deliberately hurting oneself without conscious suicidal intent, often resulting in damage to body tissue. Irrespective of the motivation or the apparent purpose of the act, self-harm is an expression of emotional distress. Self-harm is also commonly known as deliberate self-harm (abbreviated as DSH, the term used in this chapter), self-injurious behavior, self-mutilation, non-suicidal self-injury, parasuicide, self-abuse, and self-inflicted violence. Some researchers classify all forms of DSH on a suicidal continuum (preceding suicidal ideation), regardless of the victim's intent. Others emphasize the marked differences between DSH and attempted suicide and believe they should be separate areas. The majority of those who self-injure do not have suicidal thoughts when self-injuring. Although DSH is not the same as suicide, self-harm can escalate into suicidal behaviors. The intent to die can change over time. There is evidence that almost half of people who self-harm report at least one suicide attempt. In the 12 months following an episode of DSH, 10–30% of people will repeat DSH and 1% kill themselves.

DSH is more common in women, adolescents, and young adults. Incidence peaks in women aged 15–19 years, and in men aged 20–24 years. DSH is 20–30 times more common than suicide. DSH can take the form of self-injury (cutting, burning, hanging, stabbing, shooting, swallowing objects) or self-poisoning (medication overdose or ingestion of household substances). Table 14.1 reports risk factors for DSH in the general population.

14.2.2 Suicide

Based on current conceptualization, suicide is viewed as a process or a continuum of ideations/behaviors developing from mild-to-more severe forms of

Table 14.1 Risk factors for deliberate self-harm (DSH) in the general population

TYPE	RISK FACTOR	NOTE
Demographic	Younger than 35 years	Highest risk in young women
Demographic	Financial status	Low socioeconomic status and/or unemployment
Social	Severe life stressors	
Social	Living alone	
Social	Domestic violence	
Clinical	Childhood maltreatment	
Clinical	Psychiatric disorder	Highest risk in patients with borderline personality disorder and/or drug/alcohol abuse
Clinical	Chronic medical problems	

suicidality, most often including the following stages: suicidal ideation, suicide plan, suicide attempt, and completed suicide (Turecki and Brent 2016). This model of interpreting suicidality has great relevance in preventive approaches, since it gives the opportunity of intercepting suicidal trajectories at several different stages. Suicidal ideation refers to cognitions that can vary from transient thoughts about the worthlessness of life and death wishes to concrete plans for killing oneself.

Whereas DSH is more common in women and young people, suicide is more common in males and its prevalence increases with age. Compared with DSH, suicide is more frequently linked with the presence of severe physical and/or mental illness. The most common methods of suicide are hanging, suffocation, strangulation, and self-poisoning. Access to lethal means like firearms is a risk factor. Table 14.2 reports risk factors for suicide in the general population. Risk factors can be distinguished into either distal or proximal. Distal risk factors are underlying vulnerabilities that increase a person's risk for suicide anytime in life and include personality traits (e.g., impulsivity) and developmental, neurobiological, and genetic variables. Proximal factors are more immediate antecedents to the suicidal event itself and may include life stressors or exacerbation of a psychiatric condition. In addition to risk factors, clinical assessment should also take into consideration several protective factors including responsibility for others, children at home, strong social support, fear of the physical act of suicide, religious belief that suicide is immoral, and fear of disapproval by society. The probability of suicide in the individual patient results from the dynamic interaction between risk factors and protective factors.

Table 14.2 Risk factors for suicide in the general population

TYPE	RISK FACTOR	NOTE
Demographic	Gender	Men are 3× more likely than women. Male attempts are more violent and therefore successful
Demographic	Age	Higher risk in middle-aged men; larger peak in older age
Demographic	Financial status	Low socioeconomic status and/or unemployment
Demographic	Marital status	Higher risk in single, widowed, separated, or divorced
Social	Imitation	Induced by media; copycat suicides common in young
Social	Access to lethal means	e.g., firearms in the US
Social	Living alone	
Clinical	Family history	Suicide in first-degree relatives
Clinical	History of DSH or attempted suicide	
Clinical	Childhood maltreatment	
Clinical	Psychiatric disorder	Highest risk in patients with bipolar disorder, psychosis, and/or drug/alcohol abuse
Clinical	Medical illness	Physically disabling, painful, or terminal illness.

14.3 Bariatric Data

In the last decade, the impact of bariatric surgery on the risk for self-harm and suicide has been investigated in many studies (Adamowicz et al. 2016; Bhatti et al. 2016; Chen et al. 2012; Lim et al. 2018; Neovius et al. 2018; Peterhänsel et al. 2013).

The most recent data on completed suicide, attempted suicide, and self-harm in post-bariatric surgery patients come from a meta-analysis published in 2019 and based on 32 studies with 148.643 subjects (Castaneda et al. 2019). The studies included in the analysis originated from multiple countries (Australia, Belgium, Brazil, Canada, Denmark, Italy, the Netherlands, Sweden, Switzerland, and the United States) and reported the outcomes of different procedures of bariatric surgery (adjustable laparoscopic gastric banding, Roux-en-Y gastric bypass, vertical banded gastroplasty, and sleeve gastrectomy).

Mortality from suicide after bariatric surgery was 2.7 per 1000 patients. To put this rate into perspective, in 2016 the average suicide rate worldwide was 0.11 deaths per 1000 population (https://www.who.int/gho/mental_health/suicide_rates/en/). This means an estimated 24-fold increased risk for suicide after undergoing bariatric surgery in comparison to the worldwide general population. Limiting the comparison to the countries with the highest suicide rates in the world, the calculated event rate in post-bariatric surgery patients was still eight times higher than average suicide rates in the general population. The suicide attempt/self-harm event rate was 17 per 1000 patients. Based on three studies with a sample of 43,406 subjects, there was an increased risk for suicide attempt or self-harm after bariatric surgery compared to rates before procedure within the same population (mirror-image analysis), with an odds ratio of 1.9 (95% CI 1.23–2.95). Five case-control studies included into the meta-analysis reported event rates of suicide in a comparable cohort of non-surgical patients. Bariatric surgery patients had an increased risk of suicide compared to age, gender, and BMI-matched controls (odds ratio of 3.8, 95% CI 2.19–6.59). The authors of the meta-analysis suggested that the real suicide risk after bariatric surgery may even be higher than that estimated in their study. They included only confirmed suicide cases, potentially excluding "masked suicide events" (i.e., accidental, substance abuse–related, or unknown causes of death). The mortality rates from suicide were significantly higher after Roux-en-Y gastric bypass than after adjustable laparoscopic gastric banding.

14.4 Pathogenic Mechanisms

Overall, the factors associated with suicidality in bariatric patients are similar to those seen in community samples. Mitchell et al. (2013) reviewed possible risk factors that are specifically relevant to post-surgery bariatric patients. It is useful to classify risk factors into four distinct categories: psychiatric, psychologic, physiologic, and medical.

14.4.1 Psychiatric Factors

Mental health problems are much more prevalent in patients undergoing bariatric surgery than in age, gender, and BMI-matched controls. The high prevalence of preexisting psychiatric disorders combined with surgery-related changes may cause an increased risk of suicide and self-harm. Two pertinent examples are mood and eating disorders.

Depressive syndromes are commonly observed among bariatric surgery patients. The majority of patients report an improvement of symptoms after bariatric surgery. However, such an improvement of depressive symptoms may decline over time, and in some cases mood disturbance may even return to pre-surgery levels. Given the well-documented link between depression and suicide, the continuing presence or reemergence of depressive symptoms after surgery may be a major risk factor for suicide.

Eating disorders are common among bariatric surgery candidates. The prevalence of binge eating disorder is around 25%. After bariatric surgery the prevalence of binge eating usually decreases significantly together with a reduction in body dissatisfaction and weight and shape concerns. However, several studies have demonstrated that a subgroup of patients after weight loss surgery will develop or redevelop subjective binge or "loss of control" eating and even self-induced vomiting for weight and shape reasons. The psychological distress caused by disordered eating may act as a risk factor for suicide or self-harm. Another possibility is that the resolution of eating pathology leads to the development of self-harm through the mechanism of "symptom substitution." Tækker et al. (2018) reported the case of a 26-year-old woman with obesity, who initiated self-cutting behavior after bariatric surgery. The patient revealed that self-harm was a substitute for binge eating, which was anatomically impeded after bariatric surgery. She described the emotional context of self-harm: It [self-cutting] was what I used very much instead of food. Earlier, I just ate you know [...] it is this punishing myself because I don't feel that I am worth anything, anyway. And at that time, I ate because this was what I could do back then [...] It provides security, you know – that I have my razor blades. I use them and not the food – because I have gone off my food. (p. 25).

Mental problems implicated in self-injurious behavior are not limited to categorical diagnoses based on classification systems (e.g., DSM) such as depression or binge eating disorder. In the general population, childhood maltreatment is a risk factor for suicide and self-harm, independently of psychopathology (Hoertel et al. 2015; Liu et al. 2018). This applies also to post-surgery bariatric patients. Childhood maltreatment is associated with a variety of different long-term sequelae including heightened stress sensitivity, dysfunctional anger and impulsivity, hypervigilance to threat, deficits in emotion recognition, and insensitivity to reward. Each of these altered mechanisms may increase the risk of self-harm and suicidal behavior, even when the criteria for a categorical diagnosis of mental disorder are not fulfilled.

14.4.2 Psychological Factors

Bariatric surgery causes a variety of changes in the lives of patients who have gone through the abnormal condition of severe obesity for a long time. In most cases, such changes are positive and improve patients' health-related quality of life. Improvements include physical activity and mobility, sexual functioning, interpersonal relationships, self-esteem, and body image. Yet, a subset of patients continue to experience impairments or eventually experience worsening of impairments in one or more domains impacting the quality of life. When this happens, the sense of disappointment and failure (combined with other risk factors, especially depression) may increase the risk of suicide.

Mitchell et al. (2013) listed several conditions reflecting negative psychological consequences of bariatric surgery. Patients who experience weight loss failure or early weight regain continue to have problems with self-esteem and body image, especially those who know that their post-surgical outcomes are worse than others. In spite of good results in terms of weight loss, some patients are disappointed by the esthetic outcomes of their surgery (e.g., excess/hanging skin, unrealistic expectations of body appearance). Marital problems may emerge or escalate because of patients' personality and behavior changes (e.g., increase in self-confidence and social activities) that challenge previous dynamics within an established relationship. Unresolved negative body attitudes may compromise sexual functioning in spite of objective improvements in libido and sexual performance.

14.4.3 Physiologic Factors

Depending on the type of procedure, bariatric surgery may alter patients' physiology to a variable degree. Some post-surgery physiologic changes may impact suicide risk. The changes described below apply essentially to Roux-en-Y gastric bypass.

Altered metabolism of alcohol has been reported after bypass procedures due to increased and faster absorption. Alcohol sensitivity may be heightened and patients get intoxicated more easily, with associated impulsivity and behavioral disinhibition. This may explain why a subset of post-surgery bariatric patients (both those with preexisting alcohol abuse and those experiencing "addiction transfer") are more likely to attempt or commit suicide.

The absorption of antidepressant medications may decrease substantially, causing exacerbation of symptoms in post-bariatric patients who are on drug treatment for depression (Roerig and Steffen 2015). Compared to pre-surgery levels, maximum serum levels of escitalopram, sertraline, and duloxetine have been reported to decrease after Roux-en-Y gastric bypass. With no adjustment of medication dose, the risk of suicide may increase due to inadequate treatment.

In the last few years, many studies have focused on gut–brain interactions by exploring the correlations between gut microbiome, gastrointestinal peptides, and mental health. There is evidence that gastric bypass modifies the gut microbiome and changes the serum levels of ghrelin, GLP-1, and PYY (Guo et al. 2018; Kelly et al. 2019). The impact of these changes on mood and anxiety are not clear, even though preliminary evidence suggests no adverse effects. However, further studies are needed to exclude that surgery–related changes in gut-brain interactions play a role in increasing the risk of self-harm and suicide.

14.4.4 Medical Factors

Many of the comorbidities associated with severe obesity, such as cardiovascular complications, dyslipidemia, diabetes mellitus, obstructive sleep apnea, and orthopedic complications improve after bariatric surgery. However, in a subset of patients, some of these medical comorbidities may persist or worsen. For example, some patients experience post-operative complications such as diabetic keto-acidosis and hypoglycemic episodes. The reemergence of pre-operative medical problems or the new onset of post-operative complications may lead to a sense of failure and disappointment that, combined with other risk factors, may increase the risk of suicide.

14.5   Clinical Management

Pre-operative prevalence of suicide attempts among bariatric candidates may be higher than that reported in the general population. A retrospective chart review including data from 1020 consecutive bariatric candidates found a rate of previous suicide attempts of 11.2% (Windover et al. 2010). Lifetime history of suicide ideation and self-injurious behavior are most strongly associated with post-surgery risk. Therefore, pre-operative assessment conducted by an expert mental health professional is crucial for effective prevention of self-harm and suicide in bariatric patients. The guidelines of the Italian Society of Bariatric Surgery (SICOB 2016, https://www.sicob.org/00_materiali/linee_guida_2016.pdf) list a lifetime history of attempted suicide among the absolute contraindications to bariatric surgery.

Self-harm and suicide are sensitive topics that make most clinicians feel uncomfortable. Expert mental health professionals do not avoid sensitive topics and adopt a straightforward manner that conveys professionalism and makes the patient feel free to disclose culturally prohibited thoughts, emotions, and behaviors (e.g., suicidal plans, hopelessness, or self-cutting). The interview includes stepped questions that may become more specific: "How do you feel about your future? Do you feel that life is worth living? Have you got to the point where you felt you couldn't go on? Have you ever thought about taking your own life? Did you make any plans?" All the risk factors listed in Tables 14.1 and 14.2 should be assessed and weighed against the protective factors reported in the Sect. 14.2.2 above. Yet, the most important information to be recorded during the interview are: (1) lifetime and current psychiatric diagnosis, (2) past attempts, and (3) family history of suicide. There are many psychometric instruments designed to assess suicide risk. Two very short screening tools are *The Suicide Behaviors Questionnaire-Revised* (SBQ-R) (https://www.integration.samhsa.gov/images/res/SBQ.pdf) and the asQ Suicide Risk Screening Toolkit (https://www.nimh.nih.gov/research/research-conducted-at-nimh/asq-toolkit-materials/index.shtml).

Pre-operative assessment is very important, but it should be combined with post-operative assessment. Most programs focus on the first year post surgery but there is evidence to support the call for long-term follow-up, especially for patients with a history of major depression, personality disorder, and/or self-injurious behavior (Wise 2015).

References

Adamowicz JL, Salwen JK, Hymowitz GF, Vivian D. Predictors of suicidality in bariatric surgery candidates. J Health Psychol. 2016;21(9):1992–8. Epub 2015 Feb 18.PubMed PMID: 25694343. https://doi.org/10.1177/1359105315569618.

Bhatti JA, Nathens AB, Thiruchelvam D, Grantcharov T, Goldstein BI, Redelmeier DA. Self-harm emergencies after bariatric surgery: a population-based cohort study. JAMA Surg. 2016;151(3):226–32. PubMed PMID: 26444444. https://doi.org/10.1001/jamasurg.2015.3414.

Castaneda D, Popov VB, Wander P, Thompson CC. Risk of suicide and self-harm is increased after bariatric surgery—a systematic review and meta-analysis. Obes Surg. 2019;29(1):322–33. Review. PubMed PMID: 30343409. https://doi.org/10.1007/s11695-018-3493-4.

Chen EY, Fettich KC, Tierney M, Cummings H, Berona J, Weissman J, Ward A, Christensen K, Southward M, Gordon KH, Mitchell J, Coccaro E. Factors associated with suicide ideation in severely obese bariatric surgery-seeking individuals. Suicide Life Threat Behav. 2012;42(5):541–9. Epub 2012 Sep 7. PubMed PMID: 22957662; PubMed Central PMCID: PMC5670739. https://doi.org/10.1111/j.1943-278X.2012.00110.x.

Courcoulas A. Who, why, and how? suicide and harmful behaviors after bariatric surgery. Ann Surg. 2017;265(2):253–4. PubMed PMID: 27735820. https://doi.org/10.1097/SLA.0000000000002037.

Dixon JB. Self-harm and suicide after bariatric surgery: time for action. Lancet Diabetes Endocrinol. 2016;4(3):199–200. Epub 2016 Jan 16. PubMed PMID: 26781231. https://doi.org/10.1016/S2213-8587(16)00013-9.

Guo Y, Huang ZP, Liu CQ, Qi L, Sheng Y, Zou DJ. Modulation of the gut microbiome: a systematic review of the effect of bariatric surgery. Eur J Endocrinol. 2018;178(1):43–56. Epub 2017 Sep 15. Review. PubMed PMID: 28916564. https://doi.org/10.1530/EJE-17-0403.

Hoertel N, Franco S, Wall MM, Oquendo MA, Wang S, Limosin F, Blanco C. Childhood maltreatment and risk of suicide attempt: a nationally representative study. J Clin Psychiatry. 2015;76(7):916–23; quiz 923. PubMed PMID: 26231006. https://doi.org/10.4088/JCP.14m09420.

Kelly JR, Keane VO, Cryan JF, Clarke G, Dinan TG. Mood and microbes: gut to brain communication in depression. Gastroenterol Clin North Am. 2019;48(3):389–405. Epub 2019 Jun 12. Review. PubMed PMID: 31383278. https://doi.org/10.1016/j.gtc.2019.04.006.

Lim RBC, Zhang MWB, Ho RCM. Prevalence of all-cause mortality and suicide among bariatric surgery cohorts: a meta-analysis. Int J Environ Res Public Health. 2018;15(7):E1519. Review. PubMed PMID: 30021983; PubMed Central PMCID: PMC6069254. https://doi.org/10.3390/ijerph15071519.

Liu RT, Scopelliti KM, Pittman SK, Zamora AS. Childhood maltreatment and non-suicidal self-injury: a systematic review and meta-analysis. Lancet Psychiatry. 2018;5(1):51–64. Epub 2017 Nov 28. PubMed PMID: 29196062; PubMed Central PMCID: PMC5743605. https://doi.org/10.1016/S2215-0366(17)30469-8.

Mitchell JE, Crosby R, de Zwaan M, Engel S, Roerig J, Steffen K, Gordon KH, Karr T, Lavender J, Wonderlich S. Possible risk factors for increased suicide following bariatric surgery. Obesity (Silver Spring). 2013;21(4):665–72. Review. PubMed PMID: 23404774; PubMed Central PMCID: PMC4372842. https://doi.org/10.1002/oby.20066.

Müller A, Hase C, Pommnitz M, de Zwaan M. Depression and suicide after bariatric surgery. Curr Psychiatry Rep. 2019;21(9):84. Review.PubMed PMID: 31410656. https://doi.org/10.1007/s11920-019-1069-1.

Neovius M, Bruze G, Jacobson P, Sjöholm K, Johansson K, Granath F, Sundström J, Näslund I, Marcus C, Ottosson J, Peltonen M, Carlsson LMS. Risk of suicide and non-fatal self-harm after bariatric surgery: results from two matched cohort studies. Lancet Diabetes Endocrinol. 2018;6(3):197–207. Epub 2018 Jan 9. PubMed PMID: 29329975; PubMed Central PMCID: PMC5932484. https://doi.org/10.1016/S2213-8587(17)30437-0.

Peterhänsel C, Petroff D, Klinitzke G, Kersting A, Wagner B. Risk of completed suicide after bariatric surgery: a systematic review. Obes Rev. 2013;14(5):369–82. Epub 2013 Jan 9. Review. PubMed PMID: 23297762. https://doi.org/10.1111/obr.12014.

Roerig JL, Steffen K. Psychopharmacology and bariatric surgery. Eur Eat Disord Rev. 2015;23(6):463–9. Epub 2015 Sep 3. Review. PubMed PMID: 26338011. https://doi.org/10.1002/erv.2396.

SICOB (Società Italiana di Chirurgia dell'Obesità e delle Malattie Metaboliche). Linee Guida di Chirurgia dell'Obesità. 2016. https://www.sicob.org/00_materiali/linee_guida_2016.pdf.

Tækker L, Christensen BJ, Lunn S. From bingeing to cutting: the substitution of a maladaptive coping strategy after bariatric surgery. J Eat Disord. 2018;6:24. eCollection 2018. PubMed PMID: 30305902; PubMed Central PMCID: PMC6166281. https://doi.org/10.1186/s40337-018-0213-3.

Turecki G, Brent DA. Suicide and suicidal behaviour. Lancet. 2016;387(10024):1227–39. Epub 2015 Sep 15. Review. PubMed PMID: 26385066; PubMed Central PMCID: PMC5319859. https://doi.org/10.1016/S0140-6736(15)00234-2.

Windover AK, Merrell J, Ashton K, Heinberg LJ. Prevalence and psychosocial correlates of self-reported past suicide attempts among bariatric surgery candidates. Surg Obes Relat Dis. 2010;6(6):702–6. Epub 2010 Sep 16. PubMed PMID: 21111382. https://doi.org/10.1016/j.soard.2010.08.014.

Wise J. Suicide screening should be given to patients who have bariatric surgery, study recommends. BMJ. 2015;351:h5367. PubMed PMID: 26450999. https://doi.org/10.1136/bmj.h5367.

Current Problems and Future Directions

15

Abstract

As bariatric surgery procedures continue to grow, it is critical that clinicians acknowledge the unsolved issues that need to be addressed by practice and research. Many of these issues pertain to the emerging fields of bariatric psychology and psychiatry. An open question concerns the outcome measures to assess the success of bariatric surgery. Current emphasis on weight loss neglects the importance of quality of life and post-surgery prevalence of mental disorders. Another unsolved issue is the definition of psychiatric contraindications. Until guidelines clearly specify which specific factors turn a potential psychiatric contraindication into a manageable pre-surgery condition, evaluating clinicians will continue to bring the burden of deciding case-by-case. There is no general consensus on the timing of pre- and post-operative mental health care and support. However, the contact between patients and mental health professionals should not be limited to the pre-operative interview. Future directions that promise to change the current practice of bariatric psychology and psychiatry include precision medicine, telemedicine, and psychological support to surgeons.

Keywords

Outcome measures · Psychiatric contraindications · Eligibility criteria · Timing of mental health interventions · Precision medicine · Telemedicine · Bariatric surgeons

15.1 Background

Bariatric surgery is considered the most effective and durable treatment for severe obesity resulting in an average weight loss of 25–35% of initial body weight. Resolution or substantial improvement of obesity-related comorbidities are

© Springer Nature Switzerland AG 2020
A. Troisi, *Bariatric Psychology and Psychiatry*,
https://doi.org/10.1007/978-3-030-44834-9_15

Table 15.1 A clinical agenda for bariatric psychology and psychiatry

- Agree upon a standard protocol for pre-operative assessment of bariatric candidates
- Agree upon the timing of pre-operative assessment and treatment (if necessary) based on the individual psychosocial profile of the bariatric candidate
- Establish unambiguous criteria of psychiatric eligibility to bariatric surgery and list absolute psychiatric contraindications
- Make it clear which individual factors can turn a relative psychiatric contraindication into a manageable pre-surgery condition
- Define which are the psychosocial measures that should complement weight loss and medical parameters when assessing long-term costs and benefits of bariatric surgery
- Agree upon the timing of post-operative assessment and treatment (if necessary)based on the individual psychosocial profile of the post-surgery patient
- Identify the best times for monitoring post-surgery psychosocial changes and agree upon the most useful variables to measure

additional benefits of bariatric surgery. This explains why bariatric surgery has become an increasing common anti-obesity treatment. As bariatric surgery procedures continue to grow, it is critical that clinicians acknowledge the unsolved issues that need to be addressed by practice and research. Many of these issues pertain to the emerging fields of bariatric psychology and psychiatry (Table 15.1).

This concluding chapter reviews open questions concerning the psychological and psychiatric aspects of bariatric surgery. As shown in the ensuing discussion, unsolved issues involve both patients seeking surgical treatment for obesity and patients who have undergone weight loss surgery. The final part of the chapter outlines future developments that are likely to change the practice of bariatric psychology and psychiatry in the next few years. The review is necessarily selective and does not cover all the open questions and future developments that are emerging in the new fields of bariatric psychology and psychiatry.

15.2   Current Issues

15.2.1 Outcome Measures

As implied by its name, the aim of bariatric surgery (also named "weight loss and metabolic surgery") is to cause weight loss and to improve medical comorbidities secondary to obesity. In the absence of medical complications, *a primary goal of weight loss surgery and* **the measure of its success** *is the attainment of significant and durable weight loss.* (Brethauer et al. 2015: 501, emphasis added). Thus, it is not surprising that weight loss has become the primary outcome measure in clinical studies assessing short- and long-term effects of bariatric surgery.

The narrow focus on weight loss has diverted clinicians' attention away from other outcome measures that should be included in a cost–benefit analysis. For some patients, bariatric surgery may be successful in terms of weight loss and unsuccessful in terms of psychosocial consequences. For example, follow-up studies suggest that bariatric surgery patients who have been maltreated experience medical improvements and weight loss similar to those without histories of maltreatment. However, maltreated individuals often report greater levels of depression as well as mood and anxiety disorders both prior to and following surgery. Additionally, victims of childhood trauma may be at an elevated risk for psychiatric hospitalizations and suicidal behavior following surgery, especially those who are suffering from mood or substance use disorders (Mitchell et al. 2013).

The open question is what is the association between pre-operative mental health conditions and bariatric outcomes other than weight loss. We need more data on outcome measures such as quality of life, adherence to behavioral guidelines, risk of suicide, and post-surgery prevalence of psychological disturbances, and mental disorders. Recently, Szmulewicz et al. (2019) published a systematic review and meta-analysis of randomized clinical trials assessing mental health quality of life after bariatric surgery. The rationale inspiring the study was that, given the high prevalence of mental disorders among bariatric candidates, adverse psychiatric events may occur post-operatively if bariatric surgery does not improve mental health quality of life. They found that bariatric surgery improved patients' physical health quality of life but had no impact on their mental health quality of life at 1, 2, or 3 years after surgery. The findings of this study show the necessity of revising the balance between physical and mental outcome measures when assessing the success of bariatric procedures. Post-surgery changes in psychosocial and functional status may better relate to pre-surgery mental conditions than weight loss.

15.2.2 Psychiatric Contraindications

The issue of outcome measures is strictly related to the issue of psychiatric contraindications. A retrospective analysis of the reports addressing the question of which psychiatric conditions contraindicate bariatric surgery reveals a progressive expansion of eligibility criteria. Conditions that in the past were considered contraindications are now judged as compatible with bariatric surgery. It is likely that the emphasis on weight loss as the primary measure of success has played a role in changing eligibility criteria.

A good example is intellectual disability. Based on the fact that true informed consent and commitment to long-term follow-up may be difficult to attain in patients with cognitive dysfunction, intellectual disability is considered a contraindication by most evaluating clinicians. Yet, a recent paper argued for the contrary: *At first glance, the results of the current study serve to dispel any preconceived concerns that individuals with intellectual or developmental disability may not do as well as their developmentally typical counterparts, at least in the short-term. This is evidenced by the observations that the individuals with intellectual or developmental disability not only experienced a similar degree of* **postoperative weight loss**, *including characteristics of associated weight-loss trajectory, but that preoperative intelligence scores did not correlate with postoperative outcomes.* (Michalsky 2019: 1, emphasis added). An analog reasoning has been applied to patients with severe mental illness: *The decision to pursue surgery involves weighing the risks and benefits, and some patients with severe and persistent mental disorders have undergone bariatric surgery, particularly as bipolar disorder and schizophrenia are associated with increased risk for obesity. A systematic review indicated that people with bipolar disorder achieve* **weight loss post-surgery** *comparable to the general bariatric population, with no significant short-term exacerbation of psychiatric symptoms* (Kalarchian and Marcus 2019: 4, emphasis added).

The issue is made more complicated by the fact that there is no clear consensus among official guidelines regarding which psychiatric conditions merit recommending delay or denial of bariatric surgery. For example, the *Interdisciplinary European Guidelines on Metabolic and Bariatric Surgery* (Fried et al. 2013) list the following conditions as specific contraindications to bariatric surgery: non-stabilized psychotic disorders, severe depression, personality and eating disorders, alcohol abuse, or drug dependencies. Similarly, the *Resource Document on Bariatric Surgery and Psychiatric Care* of the American Psychiatric Association (Sockalingam et al. 2017) states: *The most common reasons for deferring bariatric surgery are significant psychopathology such as active psychosis (including thought disorder symptoms), current substance dependence, untreated eating disorders (specifically anorexia nervosa or bulimia nervosa), untreated depression and/or active suicidal ideation.* (p. 2). Yet, in other parts of these documents, there are statements suggesting that clinicians should make their determinations based on a constellation of factors rather on the presence or absence of any particular psychiatric symptom or syndrome. The European document specifies that the conditions listed above are contraindications *unless specifically advised by a psychiatrist experienced in obesity* (p. 453) and the American document states that *a psychiatric disorder per se should not be viewed as an exclusion criterion for bariatric surgery.* (p. 2).

The view that declines in the medical risks associated with bariatric surgery have weakened the rationale for excluding patients based on psychiatric factors (Rutledge et al. 2019) should be weighted against the data showing that, over a 10-year study period, there was an increase in mental health service presentations after surgery, particularly among those who had prior psychiatric illnesses (Morgan et al. 2019).

In the absence of a standardized guideline for psychiatric eligibility, the vast majority of bariatric programs unconditionally recommend most of the candidates and only a small percentage of pre-surgery mental health evaluations end up being denied bariatric surgery (Pitzul et al. 2014). Until guidelines clearly specify which specific factors turn a potential psychiatric contraindication into a manageable pre-surgery condition, evaluating clinicians will continue to bring the burden of deciding case-by-case, with the risk of facing a medical malpractice lawsuit.

15.2.3 Timing of Mental Health Interventions

If the role of mental health assessment is exclusively seen as a diagnostic gatekeeper to exclude bariatric candidates from surgery, the contact between patients and mental health professionals is limited to the pre-operative interview. Such a view is clearly wrong. Psychological and psychiatric care should extend through the entire surgery "journey" and includes pre-operative education and support and post-operative follow-up. The open question is: How long should psychological and psychiatric care last before and after surgery? Current guidelines do not provide clear indications.

An optimal program of pre-operative psychological and psychiatric care can last up to 6 months. All patients should be informed about long-term surgical outcomes and should be allowed to discuss their motivations and expectations. Some patients require a trial of pre-operative psychotherapy to modify dysfunctional beliefs (e.g., altered body image) and/or pathological behaviors (e.g., binge eating). Mental health professionals need time to implement all the tasks that are now required by a comprehensive program of psychological evaluation and support. A reasonable compromise between an optimal protocol and practical feasibility should take into account available resources and the risk of dropouts because patients do not want to get stuck in the psychological program (Ogden et al. 2019).

The timing of post-operative psychosocial follow-up poses analog questions. Data from long-term studies of mental health after bariatric surgery are changing prevalent views on the appropriate duration of post-operative follow-up. After an initial improvement in psychiatric symptoms and psychosocial functioning (the honeymoon phase lasting about 2 years), some patients who have undergone bariatric surgery show a progressive decline in their mental well-being. While there are clear indications on the timing of post-operative medical follow-up (e.g., every 3 months during the first year after surgery, then annually) (Busetto et al. 2018), current guidelines do not specify which is the optimal frequency of long-term mental health assessments and if there is a time limit to stop follow-up visits. NICE guidance [CG189] highlighted the need for research investigating effective behavioral interventions for patients following bariatric surgery (https://www.nice.org.uk/guidance/cg189). From the patient perspective, there is a need for continued support from mental health professionals beyond 2 years after surgery for a variety of issues that patients can find themselves contending with in the longer term (e.g., depression, body dissatisfaction, disordered eating). Although psychological support is highly valued and desired by patients, they report that there is not enough psychological input post-operatively and this is a significant missing component of their care (Parretti et al. 2019).

15.3 Future Directions

15.3.1 Precision Medicine

Precision medicine is an emerging approach for disease treatment and prevention that takes into account individual variability in genes, environment, and lifestyle for each person. It is in contrast to a one-size-fits-all approach, in which disease treatment and prevention strategies are developed for the average person, with less consideration for the differences between individuals (National Research Council US 2011).

The approach of precision medicine is already impacting bariatric surgery. There is preliminary evidence that individual genetic and epigenetic variables influence patients' weight loss after bariatric surgery. Katsareli et al. (2020) developed a genetic risk score composed of single nucleotide polymorphisms associated with obesity-related traits and found that it was significantly associated with weight loss 12 and 24 months after bariatric surgery. In turn, bariatric surgery may affect expression of numerous genes involved in different metabolic pathways and consequently induce functional and taxonomic changes in gut microbial communities (Nicoletti et al. 2017).

In the next future, bariatric psychology and psychiatry are expected to join research programs aimed at defining patients' individual profiles associated with short- and long-term risks and benefits of surgery. The critical step is to identify those clinical phenotypes that can be mapped onto molecular genetic differences and individual developmental pathways. Clinicians who are not psychiatrists or clinical psychologists often believe that diagnostic categories in psychopathology are equivalent to those in other branches of medicine: a specific diagnosis implies a distinct etiology and pathogenesis, allows accurate prognostic predictions, and dictates precise treatment. If this is not always true for medical diagnoses (and this is the raison d'être of precision medicine), it is rarely true for psychiatric diagnoses. This means the two patients with the same DSM diagnosis may have different prognoses and respond in a different way to treatment. Currently, there are various ongoing projects in psychiatry research to improve diagnostic validity. The concept of ecophenotype explained in the chapter on childhood trauma (see Chap. 5) is an example. Another promising strategy is the RDoC project promoted by the National Institute of Mental Health (https://www.nimh.nih.gov/about/strategic-planning-reports/highlights/highlight-what-is-rdoc.shtml). Hopefully, in the next few years, these advances will encompass the practice of bariatric psychology and psychiatry.

15.3.2 Telemedicine

As repeatedly emphasized in various chapters of this book, bariatric patients need extensive and prolonged interactions with mental health professionals. Logistic limitations (e.g., distance from bariatric centers, transportation barriers, etc.) may prevent some patients from adhering to scheduled follow-up programs. Telepsychiatry, a subset of telemedicine, is the process of providing mental health care from a distance through technology, often using videoconferencing. It can involve providing a range of services including psychiatric evaluations, therapy (individual therapy, group therapy, family therapy), patient education, and medication management.

Recently, Bradley et al. (2018) have reviewed the applications of telemedicine in post-bariatric surgery patients. Preliminary findings are encouraging. For example, Wang et al. (2019) conducted a study to compare post-surgery appointment adherence, psychosocial, and BMI outcomes in bariatric patients that did or did not use telemedicine. In total, 192 (96 telemedicine and 96 non-telemedicine) patients were matched on gender, age, time since surgery, BMI, and travel distance from the program. Appointment attendance, BMI, and psychosocial outcomes were not significantly different between the two groups. The authors concluded that telemedicine could help overcome geographical barriers to provide comparable quality healthcare services to more remote regions.

In the next future, the use of video-conferencing, social media, and mobile apps by patients is likely to increase at a rapid pace. The correct use of these new technologies require educational programs not only for patients but also for mental health professionals (Graham et al. 2017).

15.3.3 Psychological Support for Surgeons

Currently, the recipients of mental health care in bariatric surgery are the patients. This seems obvious, and it is difficult to accept that also bariatric surgeons may need psychological support and advice. Yet, there is preliminary evidence that this may be the case. Ward and Ogden (2019) interviewed ten bariatric surgeons using a critical incident approach to explore their explanations for sub-optimal outcomes in the context of a real-life case. Data were analyzed using thematic analysis. Some explanations reflected problems in the doctor–patient relationship and surgeons' frustration with patients' pre- and post-operative behavior (e.g., *The whole reason she was seeking surgery was to go down to a BMI of less than twenty something so that the eating disorder service would take her back on…she was seeking help, or should I say attention. They're so good at hiding things that you can't pick it up in a clinic… our radars are always switched on but unless you're a properly trained psychologist you're not going to pick subtle things up.*) Some surgeons concluded that if they had known before surgery what they know now, they may not have operated. All emphasized that they could only know what was disclosed by the patient and that they were not convinced that not operating would have resulted in better outcomes in the longer term, and many felt that they were "damned one way or the other."

Bariatric surgeons often deal with difficult patients. Psychological support and advice to bariatric surgeons can make the surgery journey smoother for them and their patients by improving communication and minimizing conflict.

15.4 Conclusion

Bariatric surgery is a complex clinical procedure causing major changes in patients' physiological functions, psychological processes, lifestyle habits, and social interactions. For that reason, optimal care of bariatric patients requires long-term assessment and treatment by a multi-disciplinary team. The role of mental health professionals is currently more important than in the recent past, and it is likely to gain even greater responsibility in the future. In order to fulfill patients' and colleagues' expectations, bariatric psychologists and psychiatrists should be aware of unsolved problems in their clinical practice and stay up to date on new findings of research.

References

Bradley LE, Thomas JG, Hood MM, Corsica JA, Kelly MC, Sarwer DB. Remote assessments and behavioral interventions in post-bariatric surgery patients. Surg Obes Relat Dis. 2018;14(10):1632–44. Epub 2018 Jul 19. Review. PubMed PMID: 30149949. https://doi.org/10.1016/j.soard.2018.07.011.

Brethauer SA, Kim J, el Chaar M, Papasavas P, Eisenberg D, Rogers A, Ballem N, Kligman M, Kothari S, ASMBS Clinical Issues Committee. Standardized outcomes reporting in metabolic and bariatric surgery. Surg Obes Relat Dis. 2015;11(3):489–506. Review. PubMed PMID: 26093765. https://doi.org/10.1016/j.soard.2015.02.003.

Busetto L, Dicker D, Azran C, Batterham RL, Farpour-Lambert N, Fried M, Hjelmesæth J, Kinzl J, Leitner DR, Makaronidis JM, Schindler K, Toplak H, Yumuk V. Obesity management task force of the European Association for the study of obesity released "Practical Recommendations for the Post-Bariatric Surgery Medical Management". Obes Surg. 2018;28(7):2117–21. PubMed PMID: 29725979. https://doi.org/10.1007/s11695-018-3283-z.

Fried M, Yumuk V, Oppert JM, Scopinaro N, Torres AJ, Weiner R, Yashkov Y, Frühbeck G, European Association for the Study of Obesity; International Federation for the Surgery of Obesity - European Chapter. Interdisciplinary European Guidelines on metabolic and bariatric surgery. Obes Facts. 2013;6(5):449–68. Epub 2013 Oct 11. PubMed PMID: 24135948; PubMed Central PMCID: PMC5644681. https://doi.org/10.1159/000355480.

Graham YNH, Hayes C, Mahawar KK, Small PK, Attala A, Seymour K, Woodcock S, Ling J. Ascertaining the place of social media and technology for bariatric patient support: what do allied health practitioners think? Obes Surg. 2017;27(7):1691–6. PubMed PMID: 28054297. https://doi.org/10.1007/s11695-016-2527-z.

Kalarchian MA, Marcus MD. Psychosocial concerns following bariatric surgery: current status. Curr Obes Rep. 2019;8(1):1–9. PubMed PMID: 30659459. https://doi.org/10.1007/s13679-019-0325-3.

Katsareli EA, Amerikanou C, Rouskas K, Dimopoulos A, Diamantis T, Alexandrou A, Griniatsos J, Bourgeois S, Dermitzakis E, Ragoussis J, Dimas AS, Dedoussis GV. A genetic risk score for the estimation of weight loss after bariatric surgery. Obes Surg. 2020;30(4):1482–90. [Epub ahead of print] PubMed PMID: 31898046. https://doi.org/10.1007/s11695-019-04320-6.

Michalsky MP. Intellectual disability and adolescent bariatric surgery: support of special eligibility criteria. Pediatrics. 2019;143(5):e20184112. Epub 2019 Apr 15. PubMed PMID: 30988025. https://doi.org/10.1542/peds.2018-4112.

Mitchell JE, Crosby R, de Zwaan M, Engel S, Roerig J, Steffen K, Gordon KH, Karr T, Lavender J, Wonderlich S. Possible risk factors for increased suicide following bariatric surgery. Obesity (Silver Spring). 2013;21(4):665–72. Review. PubMed PMID: 23404774; PubMed Central PMCID: PMC4372842. https://doi.org/10.1002/oby.20066.

Morgan DJR, Ho KM, Platell C. Incidence and determinants of mental health service use after bariatric surgery. JAMA Psychiatry. 2019. [Epub ahead of print] PubMed PMID: 31553420; PubMed Central PMCID: PMC6763981. https://doi.org/10.1001/jamapsychiatry.2019.2741.

National Research Council (US) Committee on A Framework for Developing a New Taxonomy of Disease. Toward precision medicine: building a knowledge network for biomedical research and a new taxonomy of disease. Washington, DC: National Academies Press (US); 2011. PubMed PMID: 22536618.

Nicoletti CF, Cortes-Oliveira C, Pinhel MAS, Nonino CB. Bariatric surgery and precision nutrition. Nutrients. 2017;9(9):E974. 10.3390/nu9090974. Review. PubMed PMID: 28878180; PubMed Central PMCID: PMC5622734.

Ogden J, Ratcliffe D, Snowdon-Carr V. British Obesity Metabolic Surgery Society endorsed guidelines for psychological support pre- and post-bariatric surgery. Clin Obes. 2019;9(6):e12339. Epub 2019 Sep 11. Review. PubMed PMID: 31512398. https://doi.org/10.1111/cob.12339.

Parretti HM, Hughes CA, Jones LL. 'The rollercoaster of follow-up care' after bariatric surgery: a rapid review and qualitative synthesis. Obes Rev. 2019;20(1):88–107. Epub 2018 Oct 21. Review. PubMed PMID: 30345630. https://doi.org/10.1111/obr.12764.

Pitzul KB, Jackson T, Crawford S, Kwong JC, Sockalingam S, Hawa R, Urbach D, Okrainec A. Understanding disposition after referral for bariatric surgery: when and why patients referred do not undergo surgery. Obes Surg. 2014;24(1):134–40. PubMed PMID: 24122658.

Rutledge T, Ellison JK, Phillips AS. Revising the bariatric psychological evaluation to improve clinical and research utility. J Behav Med. 2019. [Epub ahead of print] PubMed PMID: 31127435. https://doi.org/10.1007/s10865-019-00060-1.

Sockalingam S, Micula-Gondek W, Lundblad W, Fertig AM, Hawa R. Council on Psychosomatic Medicine. Bariatric surgery and psychiatric care. Am J Psychiatry. 2017;174(1):81–2. PubMed PMID: 28041006. https://doi.org/10.1176/appi.ajp.2016.1731001.

Szmulewicz A, Wanis KN, Gripper A, Angriman F, Hawel J, Elnahas A, Alkhamesi NA, Schlachta CM. Mental health quality of life after bariatric surgery: a systematic review and meta-analysis of randomized clinical trials. Clin Obes. 2019;9(1):e12290. Epub 2018 Nov 20. PubMed PMID: 30458582. https://doi.org/10.1111/cob.12290.

Wang CD, Rajaratnam T, Stall B, Hawa R, Sockalingam S. Exploring the effects of telemedicine on bariatric surgery follow-up: a matched case control study. Obes Surg. 2019;29(8):2704–6. PubMed PMID: 31134477. https://doi.org/10.1007/s11695-019-03930-4.

Ward N, Ogden J. 'Damned one way or another': Bariatric surgeons' reflections on patients' suboptimal outcomes from weight loss surgery. Psychol Health. 2019;34(4):385–402. Epub 2019 Jan 7. PubMed PMID: 30614274. https://doi.org/10.1080/08870446.2018.1529314.

Appendix: Assessment Toolbox

This appendix lists the interview formats and the psychometric questionnaires that can be used for preoperative and postoperative assessment of bariatric patients. Assessment tools are classified based on the aspects of mental health they are designed to focus on. Based on my clinical experience, the instruments reported in bold should be included into basic assessment. Other tools can be used when there is clinical evidence that specific aspects of mental health require more accurate investigation.

Psychiatric diagnosis
The Structured Clinical Interview for DSM-5 (SCID-5)
**MINI International Neuropsychiatric Interview
(version 7.0.2 for DSM-5)**

Global measures
PsyBar
Boston Interview
Short Form-36 (SF-36)
Health Related Quality of Life Questionnaire (HRQL)
Bariatric Analysis and Reporting Outcome System (BAROS)

Personality traits
Temperament and Character Inventory (TCI-Revised)
Barratt Impulsiveness Scale-11 (BIS-11)
Multidimensional Health Locus of Control (MHLC)
Weight Locus of Control (WLOC)
Minnesota Multiphasic Personality Inventory-Second Edition
Restructured Form (MMPI-2-RF)
Relationship Questionnaire (RQ)
Attachment Style Questionnaire (ASQ)
Experiences in Close Relationships (ECR)
Toronto Alexithymia Scale (TAS-20)

Body image and body dissatisfaction
Body Shape Questionnaire (BSQ)
Multidimensional Body-Self Relations Questionnaire (MBSRQ)
Pictorial Body Image Assessment (PBIA)
Post-Bariatric Surgery Appearance Questionnaire

Childhood trauma
Childhood Trauma Questionnaire (CTQ)
Adverse Childhood Experience (ACE)
Maltreatment and Abuse Chronology of Exposure (MACE)

© Springer Nature Switzerland AG 2020
A. Troisi, *Bariatric Psychology and Psychiatry*,
https://doi.org/10.1007/978-3-030-44834-9

Eating disorders
Eating Disorder Examination (EDE)
Binge Eating Scale (BES)
Grazing Questionnaire and the *Repetitive Eating Questionnaire*
(Rep(eat)-Q)
***Eating Disorders Examination-Bariatric Surgery Version* (EDE-BSV).**

Night Eating Questionnaire (NEQ)
Emotional Eating Scale (EES)
Eating Disorder Examination Questionnaire (EDE-Q)
Yale Food Addiction Scale (YFAS)

Depressive disorders
Beck Depression Inventory (BDI)
Patient Health Questionnaire-9 (PHQ-9)
Montgomery -Åsberg Depression Rating Scale (MADRS)
Hamilton Depression Rating Scale (HDRS)

Anxiety disorders, OCD, and PTSD
Hospital Anxiety and Depression Scale (HADS)
Yale-Brown Obsessive Compulsive Scale (Y-BOCS)
Impact of Event Scale-Revised (IES-R)

Personality disorders
Structured Clinical Interview for DSM-5 Personality Disorders (SCID-5-PD)
Personality Disorders Questionnaire (PDQ-IV)
Millon Clinical Multiaxi al Inventory, 3rd edition (MCMI-III)

Bipolar disorder
***Mood Disorder Questionnaire* (MDQ)**
Young Mania Rating Scale (YMRS)

Psychotic disorders
Brief Psychiatric Rating Scale (BPRS)
Positive and Negative Symptoms Scale (PANSS)
Lack of Insight Index
Insight Scale
Beck Cognitive Insight Scale

Intellectual disability
Wechsler Adult Intelligence Scale (WAIS)
Adaptive Behavior Assessment System

Substance use disorders
CAGE
Alcohol Use Disorders Identification Test (AUDIT)
***Drug Use Questionnaire* (DAST-10)**

Suicide
The Suicide Behaviors Questionnaire-Revised (SBQ-R)
asQ Suicide Risk Screening Toolkit

Printed in the United States
by Baker & Taylor Publisher Services